# slim chance in a FAT WORLD

W9-CKK-311

CONDENSED
EDITION
**Revised**

BEHAVIORAL CONTROL OF OBESITY

Richard B. Stuart & Barbara Davis

**RESEARCH PRESS COMPANY**
2612 N. MATTIS AVENUE
CHAMPAIGN, ILLINOIS 61820

# Contents

# Chapter 1
# **Introduction**

How many times have you made a sacred promise to yourself to lose weight this time and to keep it off forever? And how many times have you lost some of the weight you hoped to lose only to see the pounds come creeping back? If you are like most Americans, you are conscious of your weight most of the time and devote at least some effort to controlling your weight every year. You also practice what Harvard's Dr. Jean Mayer has called the "rhythm method of girth control" that results in what others regard as the "yo-yo" pattern of weight change—a little loss followed by a rapid gain. Not only does this pattern lead to considerable disappointment and self-reproach, but it is also actually bad for your health! The United States Surgeon General reported some years ago that people increase the level of fats in their blood (cholesterol and triglycerides) as they gain weight and do not lose these fats when weight is lost. They also grow more discouraged about their prospects for effective weight control each time they meet with another failure. For these reasons, those who undertake annual or semi-annual diets may actually be less healthy than those who remain at their higher starting weights. Because of this danger it is important for you to heed the following warning:

Weight loss can preserve your health if it leads to lasting change; but it can be harmful to your health if the losses are promptly regained. Therefore, you should begin a weight control program only if you are willing to follow it until you reach goal weight and only if you are willing to work to stay at goal once you have lost your excess weight.

Do not take this caution lightly! Most of our fellow sufferers think that weight loss is as easy as weight gain. They look for quick and easy magical solutions, falling victim to promises that they can "take it off and keep it off" if only they will take this wonder drug, eat that diet supplement which is the product of marvels of medical research, or use any of several gadgets that promise to melt away pounds in minutes and inches in hours, or to turn embarassing flab into tight, taut skin without a calorie of effort. They start these programs eagerly, enjoy a few pounds of early success (usually the loss of fluids), promptly find that the programs cannot be continued very long, and sadly regain their briefly lost weight. Spare yourself this pain and disillusionment. Choose a program for weight control that has the following characteristics:

1. It should help you to learn new, positive behaviors rather than concentrating on actions that you should give up.

2. It should help you to work toward gradual weight loss.

3. It should help you to utilize all of your resources— personal, social and situational.

4. It should make specific recommendations for changes in small steps that you feel ready and able to take.

The program tnat will be described in this book meets these four important criteria. It concentrates on teaching you *how to increase your daily satisfactions* rather than telling you which important pleasures you should give up. You will not be asked to "diet" or to punish yourself for misbehaving; instead, you will be urged to choose pleasing foods wisely and to reward yourself richly for your many constructive actions. Our program will help you develop a pattern of *gradual weight loss* of from one to two pounds weekly. Your body gains weight slowly, and it must lose weight slowly if it is to adjust physiologically to its changing dimensions. You can of course speed up the process, but in so doing you sow the seeds for rapid weight regain. Our program will also teach you how *to mobilize your thoughts, your feelings, your behavioral habits, your social networks, and your physical environment as a means of building your strength to meet the weight-loss challenge.* It will not take you to task for a lack of "will power" or "ego strength," both of which are as elusive as they are effects rather than causes of your efforts. Finally, you will find in our book a series of carefully selected recommendations for *very specific changes in important dimensions of your life style* so that you can integrate these new behaviors into a new behavioral you. Just as weight must be lost slowly, so, too, must the behaviors that are necessary for effective weight control be acquired slowly. Therefore, you will be guided on a walking tour of the many ways in which you can gain increasing control of your eating-related behavior; you will be helped to make your own decisions about which steps to take first and which to save for later.

### ARE YOU READY TO BEGIN?

Because we live in a weight-conscious society, almost everyone would like to reach and maintain his or her "ideal" weight. As we have seen, however, many of us who seek weight control do so through means that offer little hope of lasting success. Because it is better to stay the way you are than to begin a weight-control program and fail, please carefully consider each of the following questions as a means of evaluating your readiness to begin. Start the program only if you can honestly answer "Yes!" to *all of the questions that follow.*

1. *Is it safe for you to start to lose weight?* Some people with illnesses, such as Addison's disease, ulcerative colitis, and regional ileitis, should not try to lose weight at all. While it is often helpful for some pregnant women to lose excess weight, for others weight loss may not be a good idea. The same is true for menopausal women and for elderly men and women. If your doctor has advised weight loss, you are naturally free to start right in; but if you have any of the above problems, or if you have any suspicion that weight loss might prove harmful to your health, you *must* see your doctor before you begin this or any other weight-loss program.

2. *Do you have a long-term reason for weight control?* If your urge to shed some pounds is motivated by the desire to wear a size 7, 9, or 11 dress to cousin Archie's wedding, then you'd do yourself a favor by appearing at the church in your trusty size 15. On the other hand, if you realize that weight control offers a host of psychological and physiological benefits that can greatly enhance your joy in living, and if you are willing to make weight management a way of life, then you should certainly read on and follow through.

3. *Are you willing to make the effort?* Test yourself. Think of some substitutes for your favorite desserts and make the substitutions for several days. Park your car several blocks from work or the store where you do light shopping and walk the remaining distance. If you normally take a food break during the day, whether at home or on the job, try instead to go for a short walk around the corridors if you are

in an office, around the block if you're at home. Also, try to think of several *new* activities that you have long thought of doing, like reading a book on the best-seller list or starting a craft project, and spend some time in developing this new dimension of your interests and/or skills.

4. *Are the people with whom you live willing to help you?* Are you willing to ask your friends and family members to help you reach your goal by eating their snacks outside the house instead of within your longing gaze? As you go through the simple tasks above, are these important folks encouraging or berating?

5. *Are you willing to think of yourself as having a new-found source of personal power?* If you doubt you can succeed because you believe "you can't teach an old dog new tricks" or that "once a fatty, always a fatty," then you will be setting yourself up for another failure. If you think of life as a series of obstacles that always get the best of you, instead of a series of challenges that bring new strengths to the fore, then you will be ready with a rationalization to bail you out at times of stress, and you will have small chance of passing the many tests that you must encounter on the way to your goal. To be able to make the grade, you must truly believe that you can learn new habits just as readily as you learned the old, and that once these habits are strongly in your grasp they will be as much a part of you as were the things you did that allowed the problem to build originally.

If your doctor advises against it; if you have a short-term reason for wanting to lose weight; if you will not follow through with a few simple test steps at the start; if you hesitate to ask others for support; or if you are ready at the beginning with a convenient rationalization for failure at the end, then this program is *not* for you. On the other hand, if you have your doctor's approval; if you know that weight

5

control requires a slow and long-term effort; if you are willing to take some small first steps; if you are willing to make a social commitment to change your behavior; and if you recognize that you can control the things you do, then *read on and work with all due speed!*

As you read this book and take the recommended action, you may wish to discuss your plans with your doctor, family members, or friends. Please do so—they can all help! You may also wish to learn more about the procedures we recommend. You can do this by reading the professional edition of *Slim Chance in a Fat World* (Richard B. Stuart and Barbara Davis) and *Act Thin: Stay Thin* (Richard B. Stuart); both are available from Research Press Company (2612 N. Mattis Avenue, Champaign, IL 61820).

# Chapter 2
# The What, Who, and How of Obesity

Fat is the form our bodies use to store energy. We all need some stored fat to tide us over the hours between meals (or even to keep us going when we have no food for days), to surround and protect our body organs from physical stress, and to insulate our bodies to help them maintain their needed warmth. About 14% of the average male body weight is made up of fat, while the body of the average female is made up of about 24% fat. While it is most unusual for anyone to accumulate too much of any other body tissues, such as muscle or bone, many people carry more fat than is healthy for them. Fat can be thought of as the body's fuel storage just as the gas tanks of our cars hold their fuel. Carrying too much extra fat on our bodies is like carrying a gas tank holding 200 gallons of fuel in our cars: Our bodies bulge out of shape and must greatly strain to bear the excess weight.

Unfortunately, it is not always easy to tell when someone has too much fat—a problem called "obesity." Women need more fat than men, but they are not necessarily more obese than men. Obesity exists when a person's body has a greater than desirable percentage of fat, and that percentage varies from person to person. Moreover, it is important to realize that being obese—having too much fat—is not the same as being overweight. A person is overweight when he weighs more than the average person of the same sex, age, and height. But football players and other athletes may outweigh others of their sex, age, and height because their muscle mass weighs much more than the fat layers of nonathletes. Therefore, it is important for all weight-conscious people to realize that their concern should be with the fat composition of their bodies, not with their weight per se. They also should realize that the desirable weight for each person is very individual—almost as unique as one's fingerprints or signature.

Many of us use the pinch or mirror test to tell if we are too fat. Another way is to ask a health professional to measure the thickness of the folds of skin on our upper arms and at various places on our backs and sides. There are averages for these "skinfold densities" that are reliable means for telling whether or not we are obese. According to measurements made using a special set of calipers, 30- to 50-year-old men whose skinfolds are greater than 23 millimeters at the back of their upper arms, and women whose upper arm skinfolds exceed 30 millimeters, are generally classified as obese. (Twenty millimeters equals about 3/4 inch; 30 millimeters is about 1.2 inches.) Younger men and women are considered to be obese with even less fat thickness (e.g., 17 and 28 millimeters each for 21-year-old men and women, respectively), while the averages are a little more generous for people later in life.

Instead of relying on skinfold densities, the average person steps on a scale and compares her weight with the generally available tables of "desirable" weight. Unfortunately, these tables are not always the best guides when the real issue is how much fat you have rather than how much you weigh. But the tables do offer a reasonable estimate of how much above your best weight you happen to be; therefore, you will find in Table 1 (page 10) a range of weights for men and

8

women of varying ages and heights. Notice that each weight is presented as a range. For example, an 18-year-old woman who is 5 feet tall should weigh between 109 and 122 pounds. When she reaches 122 pounds, she should set her sights on her final weight goal after carefully examining her body for evidence of excess fat deposits. Upon reaching her next interim goal she can repeat the self-examination to see if she has reached the weight that appears to be best for her.

### WHO ARE THE OBESE?

Some babies are born with borderline obesity. Infants can become obese, as can boys and girls and men and women of all ages. There are more obese women than men, but the reason may be that obesity is more of a life-threat to men than to women (more obese men than women die early). Income affects obesity: Poor men tend to be lean while poor women tend to be fat; more well-to-do men tend to be heavier, while more well-to-do women tend to be slimmer. Culture affects obesity: Many first- and second-generation Americans are more likely to be obese than are those whose roots have grown deeper into American soil. Obesity is also something of a family problem: When one newlywed is heavy and the other slim, there is a good chance that the thin spouse will fatten but very little chance that the heavy spouse will lose weight. In addition, three out of every four heavy children have at least one obese parent, and two of every five overweight children have at least one obese sibling.

Family patterns of obesity or slimness have led many people to conclude that genetic factors best explain weight patterns. Genetic researchers, however, have shown that very few cases of obesity are the result of heredity, although we may inherit from our parents a *predisposition* to fatness. That is, some people have efficient bodies that seem to need little of the energy they consume to fuel their activities, leaving much energy left over for storage as fat, while others with inefficient bodies seem to use a great deal of energy to keep

## Table 1. Weight Range for Women

| Height Range Without Shoes | Age in Years | | | | |
| | 18 | 19-20 | 21-22 | 23-24 | 25 & Over |
| Feet Inches | Weight in Pounds | | | | |
| 4 6 (54) | 83—99 | 84—101 | 85—103 | 86—104 | 88—106 |
| 4 7 (55) | 84—100 | 85—102 | 86—104 | 88—105 | 90—107 |
| 4 8 (56) | 86—101 | 87—103 | 88—105 | 90—106 | 92—108 |
| 4 9 (57) | 89—102 | 90—104 | 91—106 | 92—108 | 94—110 |
| 4 10 (58) | 91—105 | 92—106 | 93—109 | 94—111 | 96—113 |
| 4 11 (59) | 93—109 | 94—111 | 95—113 | 96—114 | 99—116 |
| 5 0 (60) | 96—112 | 97—113 | 98—115 | 100—117 | 102—119 |
| 5 1 (61) | 100—116 | 101—117 | 102—119 | 103—121 | 105—122 |
| 5 2 (62) | 104—119 | 105—121 | 106—123 | 107—125 | 108—126 |
| 5 3 (63) | 106—125 | 107—126 | 108—127 | 109—129 | 111—130 |
| 5 4 (64) | 109—130 | 110—131 | 111—132 | 112—134 | 114—135 |
| 5 5 (65) | 112—133 | 113—134 | 114—136 | 116—138 | 118—139 |
| 5 6 (66) | 116—137 | 117—138 | 118—140 | 120—142 | 122—143 |
| 5 7 (67) | 121—140 | 122—142 | 123—144 | 124—146 | 126—147 |
| 5 8 (68) | 123—144 | 124—146 | 126—148 | 128—150 | 130—151 |
| 5 9 (69) | 130—148 | 131—150 | 132—152 | 133—154 | 134—155 |
| 5 10 (70) | 134—151 | 135—154 | 136—156 | 137—158 | 138—159 |
| 5 11 (71) | 138—155 | 139—158 | 140—160 | 141—162 | 142—163 |
| 6 0 (72) | 142—160 | 143—162 | 144—164 | 145—166 | 146—167 |
| 6 1 (73) | 146—164 | 147—166 | 148—168 | 149—170 | 150—171 |
| 6 2 (74) | 150—168 | 151—170 | 152—172 | 153—174 | 154—175 |

Reprinted with permission of Weight Watchers International, Inc.

## Table 1. Weight Range for Men

| Height Range Without Shoes | Age in Years | | | | |
|---|---|---|---|---|---|
| | 18 | 19-20 | 21-22 | 23-24 | 25 & Over |
| | Weight in Pounds | | | | |
| 5 0 (60) | 109--122 | 110--133 | 112--135 | 114--137 | 115--138 |
| 5 1 (61) | 112--126 | 113--136 | 115--138 | 117--140 | 118--141 |
| 5 2 (62) | 115 130 | 116 139 | 118- 140 | 120--142 | 121--144 |
| 5 3 (63) | 118- 135 | 119--143 | 121--145 | 123--147 | 124--148 |
| 5 4 (64) | 120--145 | 122 147 | 124--149 | 126--151 | 127--152 |
| 5 5 (65) | 124 149 | 125- 151 | 127 153 | 129--155 | 130--156 |
| 5 6 (66) | 128--154 | 129- 156 | 131- 158 | 133--160 | 134--161 |
| 5 7 (67) | 132 159 | 133- 161 | 134--163 | 136--165 | 138--166 |
| 5 8 (68) | 135- 163 | 136 165 | 138 167 | 140--169 | 142--170 |
| 5 9 (69) | 140- 165 | 141--169 | 142- 171 | 144--173 | 146--174 |
| 5 10 (70) | 143--170 | 144- 173 | 146 -175 | 148--178 | 150--179 |
| 5 11 (71) | 147--177 | 148- 179 | 150--181 | 152--183 | 154--184 |
| 6 0 (72) | 151--180 | 152- 184 | 154--186 | 156--188 | 158--189 |
| 6 1 (73) | 155 -187 | 156- 189 | 158--190 | 160--193 | 162--194 |
| 6 2 (74) | 160--192 | 161--194 | 163--196 | 165--198 | 167--199 |
| 6 3 (75) | 165--198 | 166--199 | 168 201 | 170--203 | 172--204 |
| 6 4 (76) | 170 202 | 171 204 | 173--206 | 175- 208 | 177--209 |

Reprinted with permission of Weight Watchers International, Inc.

11

themselves going and thus have little left for fat. (It is up to us to either encourage or discourage this inbred predisposition.) However, members of the same families tend to share similar eating and activity patterns; their similarities in terms of fat or leanness are better explained by these shared patterns than by their common biological heritage.

### WHY SHOULD OBESITY BE OVERCOME?

In some cultures (and even in our own culture at one time), overweight is a sign of wealth or beauty. But it has proved to be an expensive attribute because of the many physical and psychological problems associated with obesity. Although it is probably not a *direct cause* of death and disease, there is strong evidence to suggest that it is a powerful *indirect link* in a biological chain leading to life-shortening and life-crippling diseases. For example, the average obese adult has more than four times the normal probability of becoming diabetic, with its associated risks of complications such as blindness, impotence, and circulatory difficulties that can lead to limb amputation and coronary heart disease. The average obese adult is also less than normally active, and inactivity appears to be associated with a heightened risk of coronary heart disease. Hypertension (high blood pressure), gout, kidney diseases, and many muscle and bone diseases associated with mechanical strain on the body are all additional health hazards associated with obesity.

The impact of obesity upon life span is illustrated by statistics: For every 100 young men of average weight who die of natural causes, only 72 slender ones die as opposed to 141 moderately overweight and 212 severely overweight ones. Figure 1 shows this finding in graphic terms. Inspection of the Figure reveals that the average woman who lives to be 65 through 74 weighs about 12% more than she weighed when she was of "courting age" (a "base weight" of her 18- to 24-year average), while the average woman who reaches the age of 75 weighs only about 7% more than this base-weight average. A line connecting the tops of these average weights would slope downward, indicating that longer life is associated with resisting the general trend to becoming more obese while aging. Looking at the figures for men, it can be seen that those in the 65-to-74-year-old age group weigh exactly what they did as young men 18 to 24, while those who reach the age of 75 weigh 6% *less* than they did at the index age. Thus it can be seen that while women are better able than men to handle the physical effects of overweight, obesity appears to be harmful for people of both sexes. While older folks have a tendency to gain weight, the promise of longer and healthier lives appears to be held out to those who succeed in resisting this trend.

Figure 1   Relative Change in Weight with Age
over the Mean for Men and Women
Aged 18–24 Years

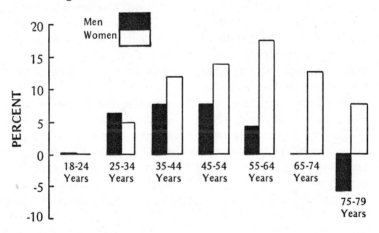

From U.S. Public Health Service. *Weight, height, and selected body dimensions of adults: United States, 1960-62.* Washington, D.C.: U.S. Government Printing Office, 1965, p. 7.

In addition to physical problems, obesity is also closely associated with many psychological problems. Overweight people are often forced into loneliness as a result of social rejection by others and an embarrassment from within that motivates them to hide from public view. Because of loneliness overweight people often tend to suffer from undue feelings of depression and boredom. Once these negative feelings develop, they set in motion a vicious cycle: Desperation is the almost constant companion of obesity, and when we despair, we tend to eat to soothe our egos, only to feel worse still for having given in yet another time.

Many social problems are also associated with obesity: Overweight children and adolescents are frequently rejected by their peers and excluded from sports and social activities. They are often victims of prejudice by guidance counselors who tend not to recommend them for inclusion in academic programs in which they are fully competent to participate; they even suffer from prejudice by health-care professionals who should be their very strongest supporters. As they grow older, many obese individuals suffer discrimination on jobs, either being passed over at hiring time or missing out on opportunities for job advancement which are freely offered to their normal-weight peers.

In summary, obesity brings to the afflicted a trinity of risks: some physical, some psychological, and some social. But all of these risks can be minimized when successful efforts are made to manage weight. For example, the risk of diabetes is no greater among the formerly fat than among the lean-for-life, and any psychological stress and social strains that obesity might have caused can be totally corrected when weight returns to normal.

### WHAT CAN BE DONE TO COMBAT OBESITY?

We have suggested that being overweight is almost always an unknowing choice. We can come into life with a predisposition to fatness, but we can also resist that predisposition with greater or lesser effort. Although few cases of obesity have a biological basis (requiring medical treatment), most cases of obesity are caused by life-style errors that can be corrected through the development of improved patterns of daily living.

The true study of obesity begins with the study of energy. Energy, which simply means the ability to produce action, is used by all living things at all times. We use energy to keep our hearts beating and our blood flowing; to keep our lungs filling with oxygen, forcing out carbon dioxide; to keep our senses active, our bodies erect, and our limbs in motion. Some of this energy constitutes what our doctors call "basal metabolism," which is the amount of energy needed to keep our vital processes going. The rest of the energy is fuel for action.

Food is the source of this vitally needed fuel. When the amount of fuel we consume equals the amount of fuel needed for basal metabolism and physical activity, our "energy equation" is balanced. At those times we neither gain nor lose weight. When we take in more energy than we need, we store the excess as fat. It is important to realize that our bodies never waste energy: We store the energy that we fail to use. Storage takes place when we are in a state of "positive energy balance," which means that fuel intake is greater than fuel utilization. On the other hand, when we burn more energy than we take in, we draw upon our fat stores, thus causing a "negative energy balance" which results in weight loss.

The number "3500" is an important one for the weight-conscious person. A pound of body fat supplies approximately 3500 calories of energy, and, when we take in an excess of 3500 calories, we gain a pound of fat; but we can shed this extra pound by taking in 3500 fewer calories than we need to keep ourselves alive and active.

From these observations it is clear that weight loss can be produced in three different ways:

1. We can eat less while keeping our energy expenditure constant.

2. We can use more energy by becoming more active, while keeping our food intake constant.

3. We can eat a little less and do a little more.

All three approaches can produce the negative energy balance that is needed. Most people who make an effort to lose weight concentrate their efforts upon diets that lead them to eat less; however, it is very difficult for many people to cut down sufficiently on the amount they eat to produce the needed negative energy balance. By the same token, it is also difficult for many people who lead normally active lives to increase their activity enough to tip the energy balance to the negative side. Therefore, it is important to work on establishing a negative energy balance by changing both ends of the equation: by cutting food intake while increasing energy expenditure. This possibility is shown graphically in Figure 2.

**Figure 2.** Energy balance

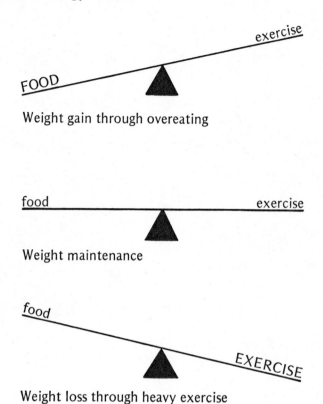

Weight gain through overeating

Weight maintenance

Weight loss through heavy exercise

# Chapter 3
# **What It Takes to Succeed**

We said earlier that overweight people are treated by others—and often even by themselves—as second-class citizens. They are berated for failing to have enough "will power" and for courting the self-indulgent, easy life. However, much of this criticism is woefully unfounded.

Years of research have shown that much of our eating behavior is under what scientists have termed "situational control" rather than subject to "self control." In a nutshell, this means that our best understanding of overeating suggests that environmental forces have a greater influence upon the amount we eat and the food we eat than do inner forces like hunger. Following is a list of five forces in our environment that affect our rate of eating:

1.  We are constantly subjected to television commercials (as many as 13,000 yearly) urging us to buy foods that we neither want nor need.

2.  We arrange our social and business lives around food by serving treats when guests drop in and by meeting over lunch or drinks to bargain at contract time.

3. We carelessly leave caches of food in all parts of our homes—witness the peanut dish in the TV room and the candy dish in the living room—and even in our offices where treats, stored against emergencies in the bottom desk drawers, are far more common than they ought to be.

4. Food ads crowd the pages of every newspaper and magazine, touting the value of high-calorie junk foods with pictures presented in mouth-watering, living color.

5. While food stores seem to be almost reluctantly stocking more healthful foods, displays of cakes and candies are everywhere to tempt the unwary into buying foods which they should quickly pass up.

The above list applies to obvious controls. But there are also hidden controls, and they may be even more of a problem than those that are within easy view. For example, it is easy to conclude that a husband's eating is under the control of his wife, who generally takes responsibility for meal planning and preparation. But research has also shown that the way wives eat is under control of their husbands. Husbands influence what their wives eat by a variety of actions, including:

1. Asking wives to keep problem foods in the house and to serve these foods often.

2. Offering food to their wives as treats on special occasions rather than offering affection, interest, or nonedible material goods.

3. Berating their wives' ability to manage their eating in constructive ways, thus undermining their confidence.

4. Paying close attention to any poor eating decisions their wives might make, while ignoring their many constructive decisions.

Few, if any, husbands undertake a deliberate campaign to fatten their wives or to keep them heavy. But many husbands have a buried fear of their wives' weight loss, which might require changes in their marital interaction. For example, slimmer wives might wish to have more social activities, more frequent sex, or a more equal voice in the management of family affairs. In other instances weight loss by wives might encourage them to move into the work world, with the result that husbands would be required to play a greater role in the management of their homes and families. In addition, weight loss by wives could imply increased competitiveness with their husbands—who are more comfortable when they exercise a clear dominance over their wives. For these and other reasons husbands and wives can exercise very subtle control over one another's eating, often leading to the gain of many extra pounds as well as to direct or indirect efforts to subvert success in shedding this extra weight.

Still another hidden support for maintaining obesity stems from many cultural ideas which we all share. For example, many people accept the notion that "a healthy baby is a chubby baby," and that adults who are thin look ill and have diminished resistance to illness. They also share many bits of nutritional misinformation, like the belief that solid foods do but liquids do not have calories; or the belief that toasting bread reduces its caloric value. Moreover, they delude themselves into thinking that so much exercise would be necessary for weight control that they are justified in sustaining their inactive lives. Finally, as mentioned above, they believe that they lack will power, or some essential ingredient that would guarantee their strength of character—an inescapable threat to their capacity to make successful efforts to control their weight.

Because of these varied forces, it is clear that any program that offers a reasonable promise of success must avoid blaming the overeater. It is our belief that:

1. Overweight is the product of maladaptive patterns of eating and physical activity.

2. Maladaptive patterns are learned and supported by life experiences.

3. Maladaptive patterns are not the result of personal weakness of character such as gluttony, avarice, or self-indulgence.

4. The control of eating and exercise difficulties must be achieved through training and skill building, not through efforts to overcome moral defects, or preaching, or any attempt to sidestep personal competence.

It has been estimated that the average person starts on at least 1.5 diets per year. Overweight people will make considerably more attempts than that—as many as 50 different tries during their middle adult years. Almost every one of these attempts is doomed to fail.

Many failures are caused by attempts to use and abuse drugs. Some drugs commonly used are intended to curb appetite; others are intended to cause food to pass through the digestive tract without being absorbed; other drugs are designed to help the drug user feel fuller after a meal than she would have felt without the drug. Unfortunately, no drug can be taken indefinitely, and all drugs have at least some unpleasant side effects. They may help in promoting short-run weight losses, but the weight loser learns nothing as the pounds are shed and, worse, she lacks weight-control skills when goal weights are at last achieved. In addition, the weight loser attributes to the drugs the strength that was needed to promote loss of weight and therefore approaches goal weight with the same sense of personal inadequacy and the same weight-producing social and environmental forces that were present at the start of treatment. This explains the almost universal regaining of any weight that drug regimens might have helped the person lose.

Other programs fail because the weight loser attempts to follow eccentric diets consisting almost entirely of selected foods such as rice, cabbage, steak, fish, or milk. These diets often pose almost immediate problems because they produce dietary inadequacies, and their followers often suffer from symptoms of malnutrition. Even those who do brave the effects of semi-starvation long enough to lose weight are more than likely to regain their lost weight. They, like the drug users, lose weight without learning the skills needed to keep the weight off. We need varieties of nutrients to keep our bodies functioning, and we need varieties of tastes, textures, and smells of food to maintain our psychological satisfaction with our meals. Because the pleasures that we derive from food are some of our more important and more regular satisfactions in life, we are not likely to forego them for very long. Finally, these unusual diets are also very difficult to sustain because they are so out of step with the normal pattern of our daily lives. For example, asking an airline stewardess on a cross-country flight for seven steamed carrots as you fly over Three Rivers, Montana, or asking your boss' wife to serve two cups of rice and one-third head of cabbage along with the Rock Cornish game hens she has prepared for the other guests certainly presents its difficulties.

Drugs and fad diets are just two of the frustrating routes that weight losers often follow. Total fasting, many traditional types of psychotherapy, and participation in health spa and nutrition education classes are other unmaintainable or incomplete remedies that pave the road to failure. As we said earlier: You need a program that will help you learn new methods of self-management that you will be able to maintain for life—methods that will promote gradual weight loss through mobilization of all your resources to take a planned series of small, positive steps.

## FOUR BASIC IDEAS
We have already alluded to the first of the four ideas that are basic to our approach: The notion that multiple forces influence just about everything we do. An analogy will help make this basic idea clear. When your old car begins to run poorly, you consult a mechanic who tells you the cost of repairs. You decide that "old Bess" has gone about as far as she will go, so you look around for a new set of wheels. You ask friends who have bought new cars recently about their experience, consult magazines that publish ratings of automobiles, read ads in the local newspaper, and decide which dealers to investigate. One salesperson strikes you as "too pushy," but another seems to have the right amount of knowledge and a gentle touch with you. This person works at the showroom where you bought "old Bess" some seven years ago, and you like the feel and the look of the make and model she has advised you to buy. The price is right, so you make the deal.

What influenced your decision to buy the car? The state of your present car, the cost of repairs, advice from friends, the facts you gathered about alternative makes and models, the influence of the salesperson, your past experience with the dealership, and the immediate touch, feel, and price of the new car were all influences upon your decision.

The same is true for eating; it, too, is under the influence of many varied forces. You may eat when you feel strong emotions ranging from joy to sorrow, so feelings are an important factor. You eat foods that you think are good for you or that will please you, and you eat when you think you must, so thoughts are an important factor. Your prior eating habits work to help or to hinder your present eating responses. So, too, do the people who are important to you and the physical environment in which food either is or is not within easy reach. Your state of hunger and other bodily conditions are also influential factors. Therefore, as can be seen in Figure 3, eating behavior is under the influence of not one but at least six different forces, and to gain control of your eating you must make changes in not one but in several of these forces. Change in eating behavior thus requires change in many aspects of your behavior and your life situation.

The second idea is the realization that eating is the result of an urge to eat, and that the best way to manage eating is to weaken the urge that produces it; that is, to deal with eating through use of the *principle of indirection.* An analogy

Figure 3 Forces Influencing the Urge to Eat

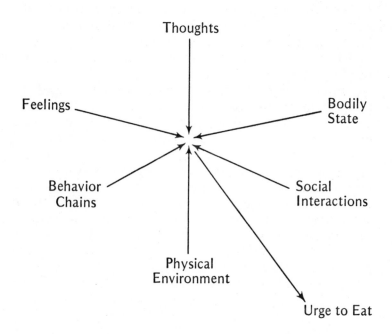

may also help to make this point clear. Engineers who build dams across mighty rivers first divert the river, then they build their dam, and finally they return the river to its natural course. They use indirection. Teachers who face behavioral problems in their classes first help students to find interesting classwork that will occupy their talents and interests, then they make specific attempts to manage the misbehavior. They, too, use indirection. Engineers and teachers both have learned that they can make greater progress toward their goals when they weaken the forces that would make goal attainment more difficult.

If much of your eating is triggered by the boredom you experience in the late afternoon before your family returns home for the day, or in the evening when television has failed to sustain your interest and you feel "at loose ends," you have two choices: You can try to stifle your urge to eat while in the grip of boredom, or you can try to find a distraction, weakening your boredom and, with it, your urge to eat. Most weight losers try a direct approach. They try to lose weight while the forces that conspired to promote their weight gain continue to rage out of control. In this book we will show you how to gain control of the urge to eat before going all out to manage your actual eating behavior.

The third important idea lends strength to the principle of indirection. It is the belief that *most of the time our urge to eat is not "hunger" but "appetite."* Hunger occurs when our body is in need of energy because it has utilized the energy available in the bloodstream. In normally active people this feeling usually begins about six hours after the last full meal and, contrary to popular belief, the "pangs" of hunger usually pass after several hours. In our society, where food is plentiful and readily available, few of us experience true hunger. Instead, we experience appetite, which is a psychological, learned urge to eat. This means that when we do eat three planned meals daily, if they are balanced albeit small meals, we will rarely experience hunger. It also means that when we do feel the gnawing urge to eat that springs from appetite, we can take steps to control that urge without eating, precisely because the urge is psychological in origin, even if we believe that we experience it physiologically.

Our fourth and final basic idea is the realization that we can understand our eating behavior best by recognizing that *eating is one step in a series of decisions;* it is not an automatic response over which we can exercise no control. For example, Mary knows that television for four hours nightly leaves her feeling flat—often mildly depressed at the way in which she has wasted her evening—and that she usually yields to this feeling by eating something that she neither needs nor truly wants. She makes a choice each night when she either turns on the TV or tries to make contact with a friend for a social evening, or goes to a neighborhood center to volunteer her services in working with the elderly, or selects an interesting book or craft project. Each of these activities would sustain her interest and turn her thoughts away from food. Even though she does succumb to the TV habit, she has another choicepoint (shown in Figure 4, page 28): She either eats or she engages in a physical activity that will serve as an after-boredom-strikes distraction—something like going for a short walk or doing a house-cleaning chore that had to be done anyway. Even then, if she yields to the temptation to eat, she has another *choice:* To eat a small amount of a well-chosen food or a large amount of a problem food. And after she has chosen her snack and has begun to eat, she has yet another *choice:* To continue eating or to leave the table and try to do something else. Thus there are at least four choicepoints where Mary could, if she chose, break the chain of events that led her to eat too much, too often.

## HOW MUCH HELP DO YOU NEED?

To manage your weight, you need several things: A good understanding of the process through which weight is

# Figure 4   Choicepoints in Managing Problem Eating

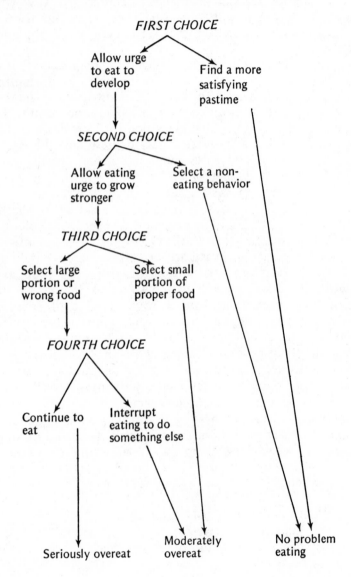

gained, lost, and maintained; a reliable method for managing your urge to eat and your eating and exercise behavior—a method that will help you to develop a lasting life-style change; specific recommendations for how much to eat of selected foods and for how much to exercise; and a support system that will help you to put these new ideas and recommendations into practice. In this book, we will provide the first three requirements. The fourth is up to you.

Weight control is not easy. You have probably made many attempts to manage your weight in the past and have realized differing levels of success. From that experience, you know a good deal about the challenge that you face. We can help to bolster your strength in meeting the challenge this time through our unique program that is aimed at managing your problem urges before you try to replace the problem behaviors with constructive action. However, as you work to put these changes into practice, you will find that some important people will support your efforts, while others will knowingly or unknowingly thwart your efforts to create a new behavioral you. For some people, then, weight control will be a team effort, while for others it will have some of the dispiriting loneliness of the long-distance runner.

At this early point in time you should make a decision about how you plan to deal with this critically important dimension of weight control planning. You have a number of different choices:

1. You could go it alone, working on making our recommendations a part of your life without the help of others.

2. You could find a friend with whom to work and share your efforts to succeed in a life-style change.

3. You could ask for the help of a professional with whom you can share our book.

4. Or you could seek the help of a weight-control group.

Many people feel that they do better when they work alone. Unfortunately, many potential weight losers underestimate the amount of effort that is needed to reach goal weight and their motivation falters when it is unsupported. Friends are useful allies when their motivation is strong, but the liability that is associated with depending upon friends is that a downward shift in their commitment can weigh heavily upon your own efforts, enthusiasm, and probable success. Professionals can serve a very useful function, but the cost of professional help is prohibitive for many people. In addition, most professionals have very busy schedules, meaning that they have a tendency to help you on your way, but not to work with you until you reach goal weight and consolidate your new life style. Weight control groups have the advantage of being relatively low in cost, providing you with an opportunity to interact with others who share your concern, and providing some accountability for your weight change, with support when you succeed and constructive suggestions when you run into difficulty. All weight control groups are not alike, however, and in making your selection you should find one that draws heavily upon the techniques of behavioral self-management, that offers a well-balanced, professionally developed food plan, and that includes recommendations as part of their program for increased physical activity (not just cosmetic exercise that is intended to create the appearance of a physical activity component). In addition, you should choose a group that will work with you in a constructive way, one that will *never* expose you to ridicule if your efforts are less than a complete success. Weight Watchers classes are among those that meet these criteria. Before you join any group, however, you should ask to be certain that it offers the comprehensive and positive service that many people find to be extremely helpful.

If you have 20 or more pounds to lose, we would strongly urge you to find some social support for your efforts. You might also consider securing the support of a weight control group, which can prove to be very helpful.

## SUMMARY

In summary, we have suggested that eating is a behavior that has much in common with everything else you do. Eating patterns are very personal and individual, and always learned. They are influenced by many different forces ranging from physiological and psychological states to aspects of our social and physical environments. The best approach to managing eating is one of indirection; that is, begin by bringing eating urges under control before making a total commitment to the development of new eating patterns. This approach is likely to succeed because, as we have pointed out, much of your problem eating is psychologically motivated and the result of a series of decisions that could be made in other ways. Finally, we have suggested that in developing skills for making these new decisions you are likely to find the support of others to be very helpful.

# Chapter 4
# **Choosing the Steps You Will Take**

So far you have learned which elements you should include in a program for personal weight control; you have learned something about the nature of obesity and how to choose a goal weight; and you have learned about the basic ideas of our program. In this chapter we will help you plan a personal course of action. First, however, we would like you to understand a little about the nature of problem eating so that you can make choices that are likely to work best for you.

## *A POTPOURRI OF OBSERVATIONS*
## *ABOUT THE OVERWEIGHT AND THE LEAN*

Whether overweight or lean, a significant number of Americans are believed to have nutritionally inadequate diets. A diet can be inadequate when the total amount of food is too small to meet daily energy requirements, or when it provides enough total calories but not enough specific nutrients. For example, compared with 1935, Americans today eat 15% fewer fresh vegetables and 40% fewer fresh fruits; but we consume 70% more pastries, 80% more soft drinks, and 85% more snack foods. Thus people of all weight classifications tend to choose foods less wisely now than they did some 40 years ago.

In part, these changes in eating habits are influenced by food advertisers and marketers who naturally promote higher markups, although not necessarily more healthful food products. Unfortunately, research has shown that the overweight are more vulnerable to this advertising/marketing onslaught. Not only do they tend to buy more of the wrong foods, they also have a tendency to estimate their food consumption less accurately than do the lean. For example, one research team has shown that overweight men and women underestimate their food intake by 44 and 19%, respectively, while the underestimates of lean men and women are 26 and 7%, respectively. The overweight are also more likely than the lean to be responsive to food when it is in plain view; to significantly overindulge in the foods they prefer while disdaining foods that do not have special appeal for them. They are more likely to eat rapidly, as though they were ravenously hungry even when they have had a recent meal; and they are more likely to define their own behavior as beyond their personal control and therefore too powerful for them to manage. While these behavioral differences have surfaced in the research literature, it is also important to stress that research on personality differences between the heavy and the lean have not been consistently reported; that is, over 70 years of research have *not* shown the overweight to be more or less neurotic than the lean, more or less intelligent than the lean, or to have more or less personal integrity than the lean. In other words, while the overeaters may act differently than the lean, they have the same level of self-management capability as do the lean. With these research findings in mind, it should be clear that:

1. As an overweight person, you should be prepared to work toward gaining control over your own reactions to your living situation and the forces that stimulate your urge to eat.

2. There is no reason to believe that, as an overweight person, you must necessarily have less capability to win this personal battle than do people who are lean.

This distinction is important. For many years psychologists believed that something called "personality" caused behavior and they attributed the problems of overweight people to their inner mental workings. They believed that:

Personality ----►Behavior ----►Consequences

(e.g., tension, low self-esteem).

(e.g., choosing foods unwisely).

(e.g., higher levels of body fat, social rejection).

Armed with newer knowledge, we now believe that:

Environmental--►Behavior ----►Consequences
forces

(e.g., food availability, lack of stimulation, and physical and psychological urges).

(e.g., choosing foods unwisely).

(e.g., physiological, psychological, and social effects).

Using the newer formulation, it is plain to see that there is a way out of the trap of overweight for those afflicted by a powerful urge to overeat.

### A RANGE OF NEW BEHAVIORAL CHOICES
Dr. Albert Bandura of Stanford University recently noted that when people have opportunities to change their own behavior they will seize the options when (1) they believe they have the capacity to make the change; (2) they

believe the change that is avoidable would move them closer to a desired outcome.

This means that people will try to develop new skills if they think they will succeed and if they think these skills will help them reach their goal. It has also been found that when people have success with the early stages of a self-management program they are more likely to persevere long enough to reach their goal. Therefore, it is important for you to choose early steps you think you can handle and that you think will prove to be of use to you.

Organized according to our time frame, but indicating the force addressed by each step, Table 2 (page 38) lists our behavior-change recommendations. The recommendations can be classified in at least two different ways. One way to group them is to think of those that (1) change the urge to eat—that is, they come before eating occurs; (2) change eating behavior itself—that is, they alter the physical act of eating; (3) change the consequence of eating—that is, they provide some positive outcome for constructive eating behaviors. This is a temporal or time-related way to organize the techniques. Another way is to classify them according to which eating-control force they seek to change: thoughts, feelings, habits, bodily state, social or physical environment. Whichever way you think about them, you will have your own classification: those that are easy vs. difficult; those that have great vs. little probable payoff. All the techniques presented have been tested in both laboratory and real-life situations; all have proven to be of benefit to most of those who apply them. The techniques do not have to be used in the order in which they are presented. We have chosen to write about them in temporal order, but you may feel bolder in some areas than in others, just as you may feel that some of the steps are more immediately valuable than are others. You will doubtless already have some of these behaviors well in hand, and you will find it possible to pass over some of the recommendations lightly, pausing just long enough to make certain that you do in fact include these actions in your repertoire.

Read each item carefully and answer the three questions that follow (Do you now take this step? How easy would it be for you to take this step? How helpful do you think this step would be?). As you can see, each question offers three alternative answers. Be very careful to choose the right answer for you at this time.

You will notice that there are five different groups of steps under the "Antecedents" category—things that you can do before you eat to make it easier to manage what you eat. Three groups of steps for managing your eating *per se* and two different sets of consequences for constructive eating are suggested. Most people find it helpful to begin with step A-1. From this record, you can often find useful methods for making early, positive strides in your eating-management efforts. But you may prefer to use a mood management, thought management, eating management, or social or physical environment management technique instead. Make your decision, using the following guidelines:

1. Omit any technique that you already do all or most of the time. These techniques are already strong behavioral assets for you.

2. Omit any technique that you think will be very hard for you or that you think will offer little advantage.

3. Choose as a first technique one that you think will be fairly easy to master. Ideally, this will be a step that you also believe will be at least moderately helpful. It is more important at this point, however, to prove to yourself that you can change behaviors you believed were not changeable than to win a major weight-control battle.

**Table 2.  Rating the Steps in Behavior Change**

| STEPS AND RATIONALE | Do you now take this step? | | | How easy would it be for you to take this step? | | | How helpful do you think this step would be? | | |
|---|---|---|---|---|---|---|---|---|---|
| | Always | Some-times | Never | Easy | So-so | Hard | Very | Some | Not very |
| *Antecedents* | | | | | | | | | |
| A–1  Keep a record of your eating to learn when you do and do not exercise positive control. | | | | | | | | | |
| A–2  Manage moods like boredom, tension, depression, and anger. | | | | | | | | | |
| A–3  Control your thoughts so that you can make con-structive plans. | | | | | | | | | |

**Table 2. Rating the Steps in Behavior Change (continued)**

| STEPS AND RATIONALE | Do you now take this step? | | | How easy would it be for you to take this step? | | | How helpful do you think this step would be? | | |
|---|---|---|---|---|---|---|---|---|---|
| | Always | Some-times | Never | Easy | So-so | Hard | Very | Some | Not very |
| A–4 Control the availability of problem foods by careful shopping and by keeping foods in special places so that temptations are kept to a minimum. | | | | | | | | | |
| A–5 Train yourself to think of food only at selected times and places so that you have some freedom from the urge to eat. | | | | | | | | | |

**Table 2. Rating the Steps in Behavior Change** (continued)

| STEPS AND RATIONALE | Do you now take this step? | | | How easy would it be for you to take this step? | | | How helpful do you think this step would be? | | |
|---|---|---|---|---|---|---|---|---|---|
| | Always | Some-times | Never | Easy | So-so | Hard | Very | Some | Not very |
| *Direct Eating Controls* | | | | | | | | | |
| B–1 Keep a record of what you *plan* to eat so you can establish guidelines in advance. | | | | | | | | | |
| B–2 Slow your rate of eating and lengthen the time you spend eating to allow yourself to feel more satisfied with less food. | | | | | | | | | |

**Table 2. Rating the Steps in Behavior Change (continued)**

| STEPS AND RATIONALE | Do you now take this step? | | | How easy would it be for you to take this step? | | | How helpful do you think this step would be? | | |
|---|---|---|---|---|---|---|---|---|---|
| | Always | Some-times | Never | Easy | So-so | Hard | Very | Some | Not very |
| B–3 Exercise careful portion control to cut down the chance that you'll eat more than you wish. | | | | | | | | | |
| *Consequences* | | | | | | | | | |
| C–1 Build in social support for your good efforts to create the feeling that others are behind you. | | | | | | | | | |

**Table 2. Rating the Steps in Behavior Change (continued)**

| STEPS AND RATIONALE | Do you now take this step? | | | How easy would it be for you to take this step? | | | How helpful do you think this step would be? | | |
|---|---|---|---|---|---|---|---|---|---|
| | Always | Some-times | Never | Easy | So-so | Hard | Very | Some | Not very |
| C–2 Chart your progress in developing new behaviors and their impact upon your weight so that you graphically see the results of your good efforts. | | | | | | | | | |

4. Now that you have learned that change is possible, look through the selections of techniques that you think will be very helpful and choose the step you consider to be the easiest for you to take.

5. Continue through the list in this way. When you feel you would like to take it easy for a few days, you may simply choose the steps you expect to be easiest for you. At times when your energy and determination are high, choose more difficult techniques that you believe will have the greater benefit for you. Eventually all of the techniques should be done and, as you gain confidence, you will find that even those that initially seemed quite difficult pose little challenge.

Take *at least three or four days* to consolidate your strength with each technique before moving on to the next, taking longer if you find mastery of any one technique difficult. Plan to spend *at least six to eight weeks* to start working on all of the steps. Remember that it took many years for you to develop patterns that have produced your excess weight; allow yourself at least a few months to learn new and better habits. Remember, too, that in this approach you will be making an effort to change not only what you eat but many different aspects of how you live. The amount of effort you put forth to make these changes will determine how valuable they are in your progress toward achieving your very important self-management goal.

In summary, this chapter has sought to help you realize that you can make a successful effort to change your eating and life-style behaviors without first having to change your "personality." It has also stressed the point that you will make a better start if you individualize your program, choosing first the techniques you believe you can handle easily and that will have a good payoff for you, and then moving on to techniques that will offer greater challenge. Finally, you have been cautioned not to try too much too soon. Instead, you have been urged to follow a leisurely time frame in this worthwhile effort to gain mastery over your own behavior.

As a means of keeping track of what you plan to do, please list, in the space below, the code letters (A-1, B-1, etc.) of the techniques you plan to use and the order in which you plan to use them. Next, refer to sections in the following chapters that are indexed according to the technique number. This will help you plan precisely what to do and when to do it.

## MY PLAN OF ACTION

First _____        Sixth _____

Second _____       Seventh _____

Third _____        Eighth _____

Fourth _____       Ninth _____

Fifth _____        Tenth _____

# Chapter 5
# Managing the Antecedents of Eating
## (Steps A-1 through A-5)

*STEP A—1   PUTTING YOU IN THE PICTURE*

We very often have rather distorted ideas about our own behavior: Some days we think we have been "all bad," when in fact we might have had only one or two very obvious slip-ups; on other days we may feel on top of the world, when in fact we have really been way out of control. Also, there may be some very clear patterns showing when we do exercise good personal control. A knowledge of those times often provides information that we can use to support our behavior at other times and places.

As we observed earlier, overeaters do have a tendency to be somewhat inaccurate in their estimates of the food they eat. Part of the problem is that the overweight, like the lean, try to maintain the best possible self-concept—often leading to inadvertent denial of mistakes. The overweight are also very easily distracted: As a group they tend to be very attentive to their environments and therefore fall victim to forces that divert their attention from monitoring what they eat. In addition, the overweight, somewhat more than the lean, often distort their estimates of food intake because their estimates conform more to what they expected to do than to what they actually did. Therefore, both as a means of sizing up our strengths, and as a means of keeping the record straight, much can be learned by keeping a written record of our eating behavior.

Record keeping can be done easily by making use of Appendix E, Daily Eating Record Form found at the back of this book. Keeping this record for at least one full week can provide you with truly invaluable information. On this form you will be asked to note for each time of day:

1. Whether you ate

   a. nothing
   b. only what you planned to eat
   c. more than you planned to eat

2. Whether you felt

   a. relaxed, interested, and happy
   b. tired or bored
   c. tense, angry, or unhappy

3. Whether you were

   a. alone
   b. with family members
   c. with co-workers or friends

4. Whether you were

   a. at home
   b. at work
   c. visiting with friends or in a restaurant

5. What you were doing at the time

   a. working
   b. engaged in an active pastime (like crafts or sports)

c.   engaged in an inactive pastime (like reading or watching television)

You can review your record each day and answer questions like the following: What were the hours that posed no problem at all for me? What did these hours have in common—dimensions that I might use for bolstering my strength at other times of day? How much of my eating took place at planned meals rather than as between-meal snacks? Did I eat more when tired or bored? When tense, angry, or unhappy? Were there some people, places, and activities that were associated with my managing eating well? or not as well?

Mr. Bronson decided to lose weight and convinced his wife to join him in the effort both because she had some extra pounds to lose and because he realized that he would find it easier to manage his weight if she were working on hers at the same time. Their Daily Eating Record Forms are shown in Figures 5 A and B (pages 48 and 50). Notice that Mr. Bronson ate a normal breakfast but snacked as soon as he arrived at work. He was fine through the day until dinner, when he significantly overate. By evening, when he was with his family, relaxed and engaged in his woodworking hobby, he was again in firm control. Obviously, the key times for Mr. Bronson to work on are the start of his workday and his dinner hour. Mrs. Bronson, on the other hand, found her troubles did not begin until late afternoon. At that time the housework was finished, the children were not yet home from school, she was feeling a bit down, and she was faced with the job of starting to cook dinner. At dinner she tended to eat quite reasonably, but then her problem flared up again by mid evening when, again, she was alone because her husband was in his workshop and the children were involved with their studies or their friends. Clearly she is in need of some different pastimes so she can find relief from boredom and loneliness during the afternoons and evenings—critical times of self-management crisis for her.

# Figure 5-A Mr. Bronson's Daily Eating Record Form

Date: 7/24

Circle the Day:
(Monday) Tuesday Wednesday Thursday Friday Saturday Sunday

| Hour | Did you eat: Nothing | As planned | Not as planned | Did you feel: Relaxed | Tired | Tense | Were you: Alone | With family | With friends | Where were you? Home | Work | Visiting restaurant | What were you doing? Work | Active | Inactive |
|---|---|---|---|---|---|---|---|---|---|---|---|---|---|---|---|
| 7:00 | | X | | X | | | | X | | X | | | | X | |
| 8:00 | X | | | | | X | X | | | | X | | | X | |
| 9:00 | | | X | | | X | X | | | | X | | X | | |
| 10:00 | | | X | | | X | | | X | | X | | X | | |
| 11:00 | X | | | X | | | X | | | | X | | X | | |
| 12:00 | | X | | X | | | | | X | | | X | | X | |
| 1:00 | X | | | X | | | X | | | | X | | X | | |
| 2:00 | X | | | X | | | X | | | | X | | X | | |
| 3:00 | X | | | X | | | X | | | | X | | X | | |

Circle the Day:

**(Monday)** Tuesday Wednesday Thursday Friday Saturday Sunday

| Hour | Did you eat: Nothing | As planned | Not as planned | Did you feel: Relaxed | Tired | Tense | Were you: Alone | With family | With friends | Where were you? Home | Work | Visiting restaurant | What were you doing? Work | Active | Inactive |
|---|---|---|---|---|---|---|---|---|---|---|---|---|---|---|---|
| 4:00 | X | | | X | | | X | | | | X | | X | | |
| 5:00 | X | | | X | | | X | | | | X | | X | | |
| 6:00 | | | X | X | | | | X | | X | | | | X | |
| 7:00 | X | | | X | | | X | | | X | | | | X | |
| 8:00 | X | | | X | | | X | | | X | | | | X | |
| 9:00 | X | | | | X | | | X | | X | | | | | X |
| 10:00 | X | | | | X | | | X | | X | | | | | X |
| 11:00 | X | | | | X | | | X | | X | | | | | X |
| 12:00 | | | | | | | | | | | | | | | |

49

# Figure 5-B  Mrs. Bronson's Daily Eating Record Form

Date: 7/24

Circle the Day:

(Monday) Tuesday Wednesday Thursday Friday Saturday Sunday

| Hour | Did you eat: Nothing | As planned | Not as planned | Did you feel: Relaxed | Tired | Tense | Were you: Alone | With family | With friends | Where were you? Home | Work | Visiting restaurant | What were you doing? Work | Active | Inactive |
|------|---------|------------|----------------|---------|-------|-------|-------|-------------|--------------|------|------|---------------------|------|--------|----------|
| 7:00  |   | X |   | X |   |   |   | X |   | X |   |   |   | X |   |
| 8:00  | X |   |   | X |   |   | X |   |   | X |   |   | X |   |   |
| 9:00  | X |   |   | X |   |   | X |   |   | X |   |   | X |   |   |
| 10:00 | X |   |   | X |   |   | X |   |   | X |   |   | X |   |   |
| 11:00 | X |   |   | X |   |   | X |   |   | X |   |   | X |   |   |
| 12:00 |   |   | X | X |   |   | X |   |   | X |   |   |   | X |   |
| 1:00  | X |   |   | X |   |   | X |   |   | X |   |   | X |   |   |
| 2:00  | X |   |   | X |   |   | X |   |   | X |   |   | X |   |   |
| 3:00  | X |   |   | X |   |   | X |   |   | X |   |   | X |   |   |

50

Circle the Day:

Date: 7/24

(Monday) Tuesday Wednesday Thursday Friday Saturday Sunday

| Hour | Did you eat: | | | Did you feel: | | | Were you: | | | Where were you? | | | What were you doing? | | |
|---|---|---|---|---|---|---|---|---|---|---|---|---|---|---|---|
| | Nothing | As planned | Not as planned | Relaxed | Tired | Tense | Alone | With family | With friends | Home | Work | Visiting restaurant | Work | Active | Inactive |
| 4:00 | | | X | | | X | X | | | X | | | | | X |
| 5:00 | X | | | X | | | | X | | X | | | X | | |
| 6:00 | | X | | X | | | | X | | X | | | | X | |
| 7:00 | X | | | X | | | X | | | X | | | | | X |
| 8:00 | | X | | | X | | X | | | X | | | | | X |
| 9:00 | X | | | | X | | | X | | X | | | | | X |
| 10:00 | X | | | | X | | | X | | X | | | | | X |
| 11:00 | X | | | | X | | | X | | X | | | | | X |
| 12:00 | | | | | | | | | | | | | | | |

51

In the sections that follow, we will make suggestions for how the Bronsons and other readers can develop the means to manage these times of crises successfully. As you read through the varied suggestions, bear in mind that our goal is to help you curb your urge to eat whenever possible. In that way you can *avoid* many eating crises. But we all experience the problem urge to eat at certain times, and to deal with these crises we will also suggest means *to escape* eating stresses with the least possible damage to your sense of self-esteem and to your state of health.

### STEP A–2  MANAGING EATING-RELATED FEELINGS

Seven different types of feelings are often associated with problem eating: Two of these feelings come from bodily states, while five are psychological reactions that generally arise from our social experience. It is important to be prepared with ways to control each of these feelings as a means of avoiding problems, and to have a plan of escape (page 60) should the problem feelings arise.

#### Hunger

Hunger is the first of the physiological states. As we said earlier, hunger occurs when the body does not have readily available the energy it needs in the bloodstream. The body signals the brain, which transmits the "feed me" message for a short time before bodily processes naturally turn to the transformation of fat into energy. Hunger is thus a *temporary* feeling that is part of the body's self-regulation signal system.

Overweight people tend to eat less regularly than do those of normal weight. They are far more likely to skip breakfast entirely, to have a light lunch, and to go into the evening hours with what nutritionists term a "caloric deficit." Often feeling that they have been virtuous throughout the day, they overeat when the evening hours arrive. Unfortunately, during the late afternoon and evening hours, natural controls on eating tend to be the weakest. For most people food tends to taste better in the evening due to a natural bodily rhythm. In addition, time schedules are less pressured, so there is more time to eat more food. Moreover, interesting stimulation and the company of others is less common in the evening, so there is little to divert the attention of the over-eater from food.

The best way to manage hunger is to avoid it, and the best way to avoid hunger is to

**Plan to eat three regular, well-balanced meals at pre-planned hours every day.**

By doing this you will be able to provide your body with needed nourishment at a time when it is easiest to control eating, thus avoiding problem eating at times when controls are weak.

### Fatigue

Many people train themselves to turn to food when they need an energy pick-me-up at times of fatigue. High carbo-hydrate foods like sweets are the most common choices. Un-fortunately, these foods do give a slight immediate energy lift, but their consumption is often followed by a biological let down that may demand further eating for relief. Most of these foods are "empty calorie" items with no nutritional value but with a very high probability of contributing greatly to fat stores.

One way to avoid fatigue is to

**Make certain that you have an adequate amount of rest-ful sleep nightly.**

We spend about one-third of our lives sleeping. People vary greatly in the amount of sleep they require; but all of us need a regular amount of sleep to keep our biological and psychological functioning up to snuff. The average American sleeps seven and one-half hours nightly; those who sleep less than six or more than nine hours often report health and performance problems.

While many people turn to drugs as a means to induce sleep, for most people these drugs have been found to cause far more problems than they solve; therefore, sleep regulation is best accomplished through a plan of rational self-management. Such a plan would require that you go to bed at around the same time every night; wake up at about the same time every morning; avoid napping during the day; make an effort to relax as much as possible before retiring; and avoid drinking stimulants or alcoholic beverages during or after dinner. The regular retiring and waking hours will help your body develop its own inner "sleep clock." Avoiding naps will help to keep this clock functioning smoothly. Relaxation before retiring will help you to fall asleep more easily and will help you avoid those painful nights of seeming to "fight sleep." Finally, avoiding stimulants and alcohol in the evening will help your body's chemistry adjust to sleep and will help you to sleep through the night by avoiding the need to empty your bladder before morning.

### Boredom

Boredom is the first of the psychological feelings commonly associated with problem eating. When these feelings arise, and when they are followed by eating, a vicious cycle is set in motion: (1) The mood, (2) Triggers eating, (3) Which leads to feelings of guilt and self-reproach, (4) Which leads to more eating, and so on. . . . It is naturally best to deal with this cycle by preventing its initiation.

Boredom is perhaps the *most common and most dangerous of all problem emotions.* It is most common because many of us lead lives in which we underutilize our potential and thus have talents and energy that are not used but that also do not disappear. Boredom is most dangerous because we tend to be unaware of its occurrence and therefore seldom take the necessary steps to combat its effects.

Combating boredom requires a form of personal life-situation analysis. In the spaces below, list the activities that you *presently* enjoy, noting how often you do each:

| Activity | How many times per week? |
| --- | --- |
| _____ | _____ |
| _____ | _____ |
| _____ | _____ |
| _____ | _____ |

In the next series of spaces, list the activities that you *would like to be able to enjoy* but are not now choosing. Also, note exactly when you think you could fit this activity into your schedule (for example, Tuesday evenings from 7:30 to 10:00 p.m.). Also note which steps you would have to take to begin each activity, from the person you would have to contact for information to the items you would need to get yourself started.

| Activity | Times when I could do it | Steps I would have to take to get started |
| --- | --- | --- |
| _____ | _____ | _____ |
| _____ | _____ | _____ |
| _____ | _____ | _____ |
| _____ | _____ | _____ |
| _____ | _____ | _____ |

In addition to these activity lists, it is also a good idea to keep handy a list or "menu" of some boredom-relieving stimulations. For example, make lists of friends you might call, books that you would like to read, or small projects that you would like to complete (even television or radio programs or phonograph records that you enjoy). Friends can offer invaluable social support and stimulation. If you have read the first chapters of several different books, you can pick up these "old friends" at times of stress. (Note: It is easier to turn to books at stressful times if you have started to read them earlier.) Projects, from knitting to completing a jig-saw puzzle, from completing a volunteer project to finishing household chores, are very effective and useful distractions. Finally, although they are passive, television, radio, and records can often be quite effective in diverting your attention from the urge to eat if the selection is well made. But beware: Poorly chosen programs can aggravate the urge to eat!

With these things at the tip of your fingers, you can go far toward relieving the boredom in your life and, with it, you can squelch the urge to eat before it's under way. Therefore:

**Analyze your life situation right now and select new, stimulating activities to program into your daily schedule, and treat these plans as having the highest level of priority.**

*Unhappiness*

A second psychologically determined feeling that often causes great problems for the overeater is unhappiness. Whether we call it "the blues," "the blahs," or "depression," this feeling is a common one that we all experience from time to time, to greater or lesser degrees. When the feeling is constant and deep, it may stem from a physical or chronic psychological problem for which professional help may be warranted. But the average person does experience brief times of depression and must learn to take these times in stride. As with the other feelings, a two-step approach is needed: One step toward rearranging life experience so that depressive moments become less frequent and less distressing; and a second step in which new, nonfood means of dealing with the blues are learned and practiced.

While these feelings of unhappiness may have a variety of psychological and social roots, very often they are the result of one of two factors:

1. Sometimes we set very high expectations for how much we will enjoy an activity and become depressed when we do not meet our expected level of joy.

2. Sometimes we become unhappy because we simply do not receive enough stimulation from our activities or enough attention from other people to satisfy our need to be appreciated.

To make changes in the first area, we should think through our expectations. Must every activity be fun or fully enjoyable? We live in a fun culture, but many of the things we must do are not very much fun at all. We become unhappy when we don't have fun, but unfortunately our failure to have expected satisfactions is sometimes the cause and not the result of our problems. Thus it is important to

**Adopt reasonable and achievable expectations about how much enjoyment daily activities will bring.**

To make changes in the second area, we must increase the range of our activities in general so that we do in fact have a higher level of personal satisfaction; and we must arrange to do more things that will be pleasing to others so that we receive positive feedback for our efforts. Therefore, whether or not we feel unhappy, it is a good idea to ask ourselves the following questions every few days and be prepared to act upon the answers:

> Is there anything I can do to bring more positive and varied stimulation into my own life?

> Is there anything I can do to bring more pleasure to others who will, in turn, respond more positively toward me?

Acting on these questions is a good way to modify the quality of your life and keep the blues on the run. Remember, when we have passing times of depression, we can do much to control our feelings by reaching out and trying to bring more satisfaction into our own lives rather than by giving in to the negative feelings that will surely grow if nurtured.

### Anger

The third problem emotion is anger. We have a tendency to eat when we become angry, as if to punish others by overstuffing ourselves. We attempt to prove, in childish ways, that we can eat whether others like it or not! Naturally, we do our social relationships and ourselves no good when we turn our anger inward and punish ourselves in this manner.

The best way to deal with anger is to modify the social situations that displease us before our displeasure mounts. One way to do this is to

> Constructively express our desires to others in order to structure situations in the most positive way possible.

This calls for assertive behavior (not aggression) in which *requests* are made—not demands. Many of us have a tendency to shrink from making our desires known to others, partly out of fear that our requests will be considered unbecoming, and partly out of fear that they will not be granted. But we

58

must accept responsibility for building our social worlds as we would like them to be. To get started, it is a good idea to imagine ourselves acting assertively and then to practice assertion in small steps by trying to achieve relatively small goals with good friends, building our skills with greater challenges over time.

*Tension*

Just as we all have passing moments of depression so, too, do we all experience tension from time to time. This kind of tension is a nonspecific worry: We are ready to take action but don't know what action is needed.

More and more people are learning that they can help discharge this tension by increasing the level of their physical activity. (We will discuss this approach and its many other benefits in Chapter 10.) Others are recognizing the great value of planning a rest-and-relaxation break at various times during each day when they know they will be able to break the grip of pressure to get things done. Meditation is still another method that has proven to be beneficial to many people of all ages. You can meditate by sitting quietly for 10 to 20 minutes, breathing in through your nose and out through your mouth, slowly but deeply, and by saying the word "one" to yourself silently each time you breathe in and out. This will help clear your mind of troubling thoughts, and will help relax your body from the physical strain that often translates into psychological tension.

Each of these methods requires practice. We must work to overcome our natural tendencies to be inactive, to ignore our need for a break until our effectiveness deteriorates badly, and to keep our tensions alive rather than working to calm them. Therefore, to manage this important source of the urge to eat, we should remember to

**Control tension by increasing physical activity, planning rest breaks daily, and developing skill in meditation.**

*Happiness*

Believe it or not, happiness joins the negative psychological states of boredom, unhappiness, anger, and tension in serving as a common cue for problem eating. Many of us have a tendency to turn to food as a means of celebration. Maybe this is a carryover from the happy-birthday parties of our youth when treats were so important. Maybe it is a result of our having been rewarded with food for our achievements by parents and other relatives. Maybe it is just a generalization of feelings of happiness with an accomplishment to the satisfaction we often feel while we are eating. Whatever it is, this is the least necessary of all mood-triggered eating. We must simply learn to train ourselves to savor the fruits of our efforts without reinforcing ourselves with food. We can tell others about what we have accomplished, or we can use the energy derived from achievement to fuel our moving out into another activity. Whatever we do, it is important that we train ourselves to turn toward nonfood activities at times when our spirits and our energy levels are high.

*An Escape Procedure*

Thus far we have talked about various ways to avoid problem eating that results from physiological and psychological feelings. At times, however, we will all feel hungry or fatigued, bored, unhappy, angry, or tense. But when these feelings come, we need dependable ways to respond without overeating. Many of us have trained ourselves to turn to food when strong emotions occur so that eating has become a high-strength habit for us at times of arousal. Just as we learned to rely on eating so, too, can we train ourselves to learn a different and more constructive response at these times.

Three different steps have proven useful as escape procedures for many people. They are:

1. When problem emotions arise, turn immediately to

some pleasant, stimulating activity.

2. When problem emotions arise, engage in some comfortable but moderately vigorous physical activity.

3. If you must eat when problem emotions arise, plan to take a small amount of a food that is not your favorite.

The value of stimulating activities is obvious: They can help divert your attention from your troubles long enough to recoup your psychological resources. The value of physical activity lies in the fact that it is a very dependable way of increasing your vibrance and energy. It also helps provide a worthwhile diversion that can take your attention away from your cares. The value of planning a snack in advance is that it increases the likelihood that you will stay within your eating plan at times of crisis. The value of choosing a nonpreferred food is that you will naturally eat less of foods that are not your favorites than you will of foods that you dearly love. Many of us reward ourselves for having problem feelings by using these feelings as tickets of admission to the pantry shelf where we store our treats—one of the worst kinds of personal malprogramming we can undertake.

### A-3  THINKING YOUR WAY TO CONSTRUCTIVE ACTION

Our thoughts usually precede our actions. In other words, most of the time we have an idea about what to do before we act in a particular way. Thus, if our thoughts are negative, so, too, will our actions be negative. Fortunately, however, positive thoughts often lead to positive actions, and therein lies one source of hope for our success.

Many overweight people have a tendency to think in negative terms. For example, they tend to think that they are either all good or all bad, with no shades of fairly good or a little bad, meaning that when a mistake is made all of the good is forgotten. Many people also tend to think more about negative events and obstacles in their lives than about positive experiences and opportunities. In addition, many people are more concerned with terminal thinking about why things happened than they are with thinking about how matters could be improved. When these mistakes are made—all-or-nothing thinking, negative rather than positive stress, and concern with why rather than how things happen—the result is often negative moods and negative actions. Therefore, it is very important to start yourself with the right ideas by planning to *review the expected events of each day. Then:*

1. Imagine yourself acting in the most positive way possible so that you can enjoy the most positive possible outcome; and

2. Plan your actions so that you can translate each anticipated obstacle into an opportunity for you to take small constructive steps toward your goal.

Imaging your taking positive action will help you develop the "feel" for such action in much the same way successful athletes visualize their hitting a home run or clearing the high bar before they start to act. Planning small steps rather than impossible giant steps, and planning positive rather than negative actions will further prompt you to act in a manner that is most likely to result in your accomplishing all you set out to do.

### A-4 CONTROLLING THE AVAILABILITY OF DESIRABLE AND PROBLEM FOODS

As the title of our book suggests, we all live in a "fat world," a world that surrounds us with reminders of foods we don't want and should not eat. Weight management therefore pits us in a constant struggle between our efforts to follow an eating plan and the efforts of food manufacturers, marketers, and advertisers to influence us to eat their problem foods.

You can begin the process of prudent buying by training yourself to find the flaws or, better still, to ignore entirely the television commercials and food ads intended to heighten your appetite for problem foods. The true test, however, comes when you enter the market to make your purchases. There you will find problem foods prominently displayed, often with "cents-off" signs to lure you off your guard. You will also find foods dressed up in eye-appealing packages that cost the consumer billions of dollars—money spent to build the urge to take home what you would not otherwise buy. This packaging is termed "point-of-sale advertising," and it is as important to resist the cellophane-wrapped goodies or those not-so-appealing treats with pictures printed on the package as it is to resist the ads to which you have been repeatedly overexposed. To help you make prudent choices at the market, there are several things you can do:

1. Prepare a list of needed items before you enter the store and buy *nothing* that is not on your list.

2. Shop after you have eaten a full meal.

3. Avoid browsing! Walk only through the aisles that stock the foods you need.

By focusing on needed items you will reduce your exposure to problem foods. Shopping after a full meal will allow you to make purchases when your resistance is greatest and will minimize chances that you will buy more than you need now. This will lessen the chance that you will eat more than you want later. Finally, confining your shopping to the necessary aisles will keep you safely distant from the sweets and other treats you find hard to resist.

If you shop for a family, you may feel impelled to buy foods that pose problems for you but that are desired by others. Bear in mind that your spouse and children can probably benefit from reducing their consumption of sweets even if their weight is normal, and that they can always buy their treats outside the home so that you do not have to set different traps for yourself on each and every pantry shelf. However, if you do buy problem foods or if you have overeating problems with basic food items like bread, there is still a great deal you can do to control your urge to eat:

1. Buy as many nonproblem foods as you can.

2. If you must buy problem foods, buy them in a form that requires the greatest possible level of preparation in the smallest possible portions.

3. Store all foods in covered containers that are kept only in the kitchen.

If you have nonproblem foods available—like fresh vegetables and fruits—you will be more likely to turn to these than to problem foods. If you must buy rolls, buy them in bake-and-serve form so that some effort must go into their preparation; toast bread rather than eating it untoasted. Do anything you can to *lengthen the chain of behaviors between the decision to eat and the actual process of eating* because each step in the chain is another choicepoint at which you can decide to turn away from food. Also, while buying foods in portion servings is more expensive, it reduces the likelihood that you will eat more than a single portion. For example, dry breakfast cereals in small single-portion servings are preferable to the less expensive, giant-sized boxes. Why? Because the amount you eat is premeasured for you, and that reduces the likelihood that you will eat excessively. Finally, storing all food in covered containers that are out of sight in the kitchen reduces temptation and frees you from having to inhibit the urge to snack throughout the house.

64

## A–5  RETRAIN YOUR URGE TO EAT

Most of us are quite careless about our eating urges. As noted above, we actually train ourselves to eat when we have problem feelings. We also train ourselves to turn to food when we engage in certain activities or enter certain places. Just as surely as Pavlov trained his dogs to salivate when the bell that accompanied feeding was rung, so, too, do we tend to train our fancies to turn to food when we constantly eat while watching television, reading a book, watching a movie, or settling down to work. In the same way, if we eat sweets in the living room, bedroom, den, or car, we will come to feel appetite whenever we enter each room or start to drive to work. Each of these is what psychologists call a "conditioned reaction." But any reaction that has been conditioned can also be "deconditioned," and that is the step you should now take.

By looking at the Daily Eating Record you have kept you will find some clues as to where your self-conditioning has gone astray. Are there certain people, places, and activities that are associated with your problem eating? If so, plan to take the needed action. You must:

1.  Decide to make eating a "pure" experience by engaging in no activities while you eat other than socializing with family or friends.

2.  Do all of your eating in the kitchen or dining room, and then only while sitting down at your personal place at the table or counter.

By interrupting the connection between eating and activities like watching television or reading, you can reduce the chances that you will feel the urge to eat whenever the tube comes on, or whenever you open a book. By confining your eating to the kitchen or dining room, you will eventually free yourself from the urge to eat just because you pass through a different part of your house.

You can also take one further step in this regard—a kind of master step. We change places and activities many times each day and our routines are not always constant, but time is a constant dimension of our human experience. If we can learn to "eat by the clock," we can train ourselves to avoid preoccupation with food at all but a few selected hours of the day; therefore, the third step in this sequence is:

3. Plan to eat your meals and snacks, if you must have them, only at preselected times of the day, following the same schedule every day.

This way you will think of food only at 8:00 a.m., 12:30 p.m., 3:30 p.m., and 6:30 p.m., or whatever hours you choose for yourself; and you will eventually be freed from preoccupation to eat at other times of the day or night.

These, then, are some of the techniques you can use to manage the antecedents of your eating. Most will help you avoid or minimize the urge to eat, while others will help you escape the urges that do arise. The key to the techniques is *planning based on self-knowledge.* The plans are *positive actions* taken in *small steps;* the self-knowledge is developed through keeping a record of the conditions under which you eat wisely or imprudently so that you can learn when your strengths are high and when you face the need for new constructive action.

# Chapter 6
# **Managing Your Actual Eating Behavior**
## (Steps B-1 through B-3)

When you take the antecedent steps outlined in the last chapter, you can greatly diminish your urge to eat; you can restrain eating impulses and make them easier to manage when they do occur. Naturally, we must all eat something every day, and therefore we must all have the skills necessary to manage what we eat. We suggest three clusters of techniques for bringing this control about.

### B–1 PLAN AND RECORD
### WHAT YOU EAT BEFORE YOU EAT IT

Research reviewed earlier showed that both the obese and the lean tend to underestimate what they eat. While our eyes may be bigger than our stomachs, our recall is almost always smaller than our actual behavior. This means that keeping a *written* record of our food intake is necessary if we are to have an accurate picture of how much we eat.

Once we have decided to keep a record, our next choice is between making notes before or after we eat. Keeping records before eating helps to make a commitment to a specific amount of food and increases the likelihood that we will use our best judgment in making food choices; keeping records after eating may lead to slightly greater accuracy in

67

noting our intake. Because self-moderation is more important in this effort than complete accuracy, there is good reason to make recordings *before* eating and to depend upon the eating record as an aid in planning food intake.

In addition to its value in planning, use of the Daily Eating Record Form also provides a source of "feedback" about how much you have eaten and how much more you will be able to eat. We all need feedback about our own behavior if we are to be able to realize our plans, and this source of information is invaluable to anyone concerned about weight management. For example, when you walk along the sidewalk, you constantly attend to the whereabouts of other people, obstructions, and vehicles. You should no more walk along the sidewalk with your eyes closed (so that you have no feedback) than you should work on eating management without a dependable source of feedback to help you know both what you are doing and what you should do next. For this purpose, special cards are provided at the back of this book where their use will be explained. Please make a commitment to yourself to use these records daily for the first several weeks of your self-management program, and then at least once per week thereafter as a means of self-checking your continuing success.

### B–2 MANAGE THE RATE OF YOUR EATING TO INCREASE SATISFACTION WHILE HOLDING QUANTITIES DOWN

Satisfaction with food or "satiety" is your body's *chemical* response to the nourishment it receives. When you put food into your mouth, the food-processing mechanisms of your body begin their work immediately. For example, digestion of carbohydrates begins while the food is still in your mouth, although the process of breaking down other foods into their component parts for absorption by your body does not begin until the food reaches your stomach or small intestine. It takes time for this chemical reaction to be completed, for the resulting compounds to be absorbed into your bloodstream, for the blood to carry these chemical messages to one segment of your brain, and for this segment to relay the "I've had enough" message to another segment of your brain that registers your conscious awareness of your bodily state. Currently, the best estimate is that the time needed to move from the first bite to the satiety message is about 20 minutes. It is as important for you to remember "20 minutes" as it is for you to remember that you will tend to lose one pound of fat for every 3500 fewer calories that you consume, or for every 3500 extra calories that you burn in activity.

As we said earlier, research has shown that the overweight tend to eat as though they were hungry at all times. That is, they tend to take large mouthfuls of food rapidly, with little "toying" with their food. In contrast, lean people tend to take lesser amounts of food into their mouths with each bite, tend to chew slowly, and tend to pause longer between mouthfuls. Since the 20-minute satiety delay is constant no matter how much food is eaten, the overweight have a tendency to eat much more food before they experience satiety than do the lean. When they succeed in slowing the rate of their eating, the overweight can painlessly reduce the amount they eat because satiety tends to be no greater when eating has been excessive than when the diner has eaten a modest, appropriate meal.

This line of reasoning supports two of the three time-related steps that have proven very helpful in overeaters' efforts to curb their excesses:

1. Pause for at least two to five minutes *before* beginning to eat.

2. Slow your rate of eating by placing utensils on your plate after every mouthful, not picking them up again until the food has been swallowed.

There are three important reasons for pausing for two to five minutes before beginning to eat. First, this pause will help prove that you *do* have the ability to control your eating despite the many times in the past that you have probably told yourself you "can't" control what you eat or the way you eat. Second, this pause will give you a moment to think about your plans for the meal so that you will have some clearly stated behavioral objectives, such as "eat slowly," or "take no seconds." Third, the pause will give others with whom you are eating a chance to get a head start, thus increasing the likelihood that you will all finish the meal at the same time. When you, who may normally eat faster, finish normal helpings first, you may feel considerable pressure to continue to eat because food is available and because others are still eating.

The logic of replacing your utensils on your plate between mouthfuls is that it will necessarily lead to a slowing of your rate of food consumption and this, in turn, will help you build a more natural eating rhythm. When you are able to extend the time it takes you to eat a normal first helping to close to 20 minutes, you will find increasing satisfaction with what you eat without overeating. As an added benefit, as you slow your rate of eating, you will chew your food better and make it more digestible; and you are also likely to find that you enjoy the food you eat more because you can savor its taste and texture.

The third possible manipulation of time is also intended to help shield you from overeating. It is:

3. Wait at least 10 minutes before starting to eat any unplanned snack.

As mentioned earlier, following the recommendations for managing the antecedents of your eating will help minimize your urge to eat, but no prevention program is perfect and you, like all of us, are likely to have occasional urges to eat inappropriately. At these times you can give in to the eating urge immediately, and thereby lose the battle before it is begun. Or you can wait at least 10 minutes before you start eating any unplanned snack, thereby giving yourself an opportunity to be diverted and perhaps avoid the snack entirely. You can fill the time by engaging in some physical activity which may provide the stimulation you craved, or by reading a few chapters in a book, calling a friend, putting a few more pieces in a jig-saw puzzle, or any other distracting activity. Doing these things helps a great many people to short circuit the eating cycle before any damage is done.

## B–3 EXERCISE CARE IN CHOOSING PORTIONS OF THE PROPER FOODS

In addition to managing the rate of your eating, you can also control the size of the portions that you eat and thereby greatly reduce the amount you eat. There are three steps you can take to make this important task easier to accomplish:

1. Measure every portion you take.

2. Make normal portions appear to be large.

3. Make second helpings difficult to get.

The value of the first step has been shown by research which demonstrated that both the overweight and the lean are often *inaccurate* in judging the size of portions of different kinds of food, generally tending to *underestimate* portion sizes. If you follow an eating plan but underestimate portion size by 20% or more, you can all but destroy the potential value of the program you are following. Therefore, an inexpensive food scale, measuring cup, spoon, and ruler can all be highly valuable aids in helping you to eat the right amount of all the foods you ought to eat (see also Appendix G, Equivalents by Volume).

You can make portions appear large by measuring the proper amounts and serving them on a 7" salad plate instead of a 9" dinner plate. This is important because much of our feeling of satisfaction comes from what we think we have eaten, independent of how much we actually ate. This conclusion is the result of research done in several laboratories in which people were given liquid meals to drink, some high in caloric value and some low. Some were told that the liquids were high in value when they were actually low; and some were told that the liquids were low when they actually contained relatively more caloric density. The result: Those who thought they had the rich liquid felt more satisfied than those who thought they had the weaker liquid, whether or not their belief was correct. You can use this same principle to your own advantage by helping yourself see smaller portions as being larger.

The same principle can also work to your advantage in the third step: When second helpings are in plain view and easy to reach, you are very much more likely to have an appetite for this extra food. On the other hand, when food is out of sight, it is very likely to be out of mind! Also, you are offered more choicepoints since you have to take steps to obtain more food. Therefore, keeping serving dishes off the table (better still, in the kitchen, if you are eating in the dining room) can be a useful tool in your self-management efforts. You do not have to confine this technique to your own home. For example, when eating in restaurants you might ask the waiter to remove the rolls you do not plan to eat; and you might choose to order a fixed portion from the menu rather than eating from a smorgasbord. In the same vein, moving away from food at parties can make it easier to meet the eating-management challenge when you are visiting because the less contact you have with food, the easier it will be for you to control what you eat.

As mentioned earlier, it is very important to make certain you always have on hand the foods you plan to eat. Naturally, it will be easier for you to eat as planned when the needed foods are easily available. Many weight losers triple their struggle when they do not have a supply of desirable foods on hand but do have some problem foods on the problem shelves. For all of us, some foods are more tempting than others, and if you have these problem foods available, but not those you plan to eat, you are surely stacking the odds against your efforts if effective self-management is your goal.

In conclusion, we have suggested a variety of techniques that you can use to manage exactly what you eat. Beginning with a before-eating record and moving on to management of both the temporal dimensions of your eating and the visual cues for eating, you can build a great deal of direct control into your eating behavior. The steps will be easier if they are taken in the context of managing the antecedents (Chapter 5) and the consequences (Chapter 7) of your eating. However, many people take these steps first and learn that they can, in fact, meet a challenge they always thought was too great for them. This lesson provides the encouragement needed to take control of the before-and-after steps in successful self-management.

# Chapter 7
# Managing the Consequences of Successful Eating Behavior
## (Steps C-1 through C-2)

It is as important to make certain that your payoff will follow your personal successes as it is to work to bring about success. These payoff experiences are the events that make self-management worth the effort! There are two ways that you can build these payoffs into your program: by developing your resources for social support, and by utilizing a feedback system.

### C–1 BUILDING SOCIAL SUPPORT FOR YOUR SUCCESSFUL EFFORTS

Many of us would like to think we can meet all challenges single-handedly. Indeed, there is a strong independence value in our society that has long recognized the accomplishments of the lone explorer, the unaided flight across an ocean, and successful efforts to "pull oneself up by the bootstraps." In reality, however, even those individual achievers tend to have invaluable backing of others before and after, although not during, their achievements. You, too, will benefit greatly from the support you receive from others in your efforts to manage your eating and to change your patterns of physical activity.

We live in highly social worlds—even those who physically live alone. We have extended family members like parents, sisters and brothers, aunts and uncles, nephews and nieces; we have friends, neighbors, and co-workers; we have the option of joining groups that form specifically to support our efforts to gain self-mastery skills. These are not automatic networks; to make them work for us, we must take steps to set their processes in motion. Therefore, you should make a commitment to include others in your planning by taking the following steps:

1. Identify the people who are most likely to be of help to you.

2. Inform them about your specific plans.

3. Enlist their positive support.

Choose one or more of the following as helpers: family members, friends, co-workers, or a weight-control group such as Weight Watchers. As noted earlier, family members have a great influence upon your psychological state of being, your eating, and your health. Unfortunately, members of your family do not necessarily always work to help you achieve your goals, and you may have to work toward redirecting their efforts. They, like many of your friends and co-workers, may have a stake in seeing you stay the way you are. On the other hand, weight-control groups are always change oriented and can provide consistent, sympathetic, and informed support. Even if you do receive help from family members, you may gain added strength from seeking the help of friends, co-workers, and focal groups.

Once you have selected those people you would like to join your team, let them know that it is important for you to gain control of your weight, both in order to improve your health and appearance and to give you the invaluable psychological lift that comes from achieving success in self-management. Tell them exactly what you plan to do (giving them a copy of this book is an effective way to communicate this information); then ask their counsel on how they can best assist you.

You can get help from others in three important ways: They can set a good example; they can remind you about your goals; and they can pay close attention to you when you achieve your daily goals. By not eating problem foods in careless ways, they can serve as good models for you and can, at the same time, help minimize your temptations. By gentle reminders they can help keep your energies focused on the self-management tasks you select. And by attending to you when you succeed, they can give you their most powerful asset: interest in you and your achievements. Unfortunately, many well-meaning relatives and friends often ignore positives and nag about negatives; the result is that you are far more likely to be provoked into anger and overeating than into taking constructive steps. Therefore, you must caution your would-be helpers that they must *ignore your slips* and *recognize your successes clearly* if they are to be of help to you.

You can also build some material payoffs into your social-support system if you wish. You can do this by asking others to help you to systematically reward yourself for successful behavior. For example, you might take the course set by many successful weight-losers and use a "token system," which is a way of giving yourself tokens or points for each achievement. You can then make the payoff following your earning a given number of tokens. The things which you do may be worth a different number of tokens. For example, the woman in Figure 6 (page 78) earned 3 points for following a meal plan for one meal and 100 points for following it for 21 meals in a row. She could then choose the way to spend her hard-earned points from a list of things she wanted, called a "menu." She could, for example, buy an extra 15 minutes of conversation with her husband for 3 tokens, or an extra 3 hours of baby-sitting for 25. Using Figure 6 as a guide, try to work out a token system for yourself. Make sure you talk it over with all of the people helping—your mate, friends, co-workers, or others. You will be surprised at how willing these people will be to help you get payoffs for what you do, and your success can become their pleasure because they will have had a hand in helping you earn it.

**Figure 6  Token Reinforcement Menu**

| Responses Earning Tokens | | |
| --- | --- | --- |
| Response | Amount | Number of Tokens |
| Follow diet | 1 meal | 3 |
| Follow diet | 3 consecutive meals | 12 |
| Follow diet | 7 consecutive days | 100 |
| Walk | 1 block | .5 |
| Walk | 6 blocks | 6 |
| Walk | 20 blocks | 25 |
| Redemption Value of Tokens | | |
| Item | | Number of Tokens |
| Extra 15 min. conversation | | 3 |
| Extra evening out | | 25 |
| Extra baby sitter for 3 hours during day | | 25 |
| $2 surprise | | 100 |
| New dress | | 500 |
| Special weekend trip | | 1500 |

Whether you keep the support system informal, join a group, or set up a token system, remember to keep two things in mind:

1. You can always benefit from receiving social support.

2. You can't be spoiled by support because you can use all you can get!

## C–2  CHART YOUR PROGRESS

Just as you can benefit greatly from feedback about what you eat so, too, can you gain from feedback about your overall progress. The ultimate payoff for your good efforts will be a change in your weight. Weight may not, however, change immediately, and it will almost certainly change irregularly. Most people lose fluids quickly when they begin a weight-control program, but their losses level off after a few weeks. They may lose more weight some weeks than others, and may actually record weight gains from time to time. These plateaus and gains are caused by a number of different things: premenstrual fluid retention in women; extra fluid retention attributable to a slight increase in the saltiness of foods eaten; changes in level of activity; and, of course, changes in the amount of food eaten. It is important to take these expected irregularities in your stride, using them as information, not punishment. Keep up what you are doing, even if you do not appear to be losing weight because weight will eventually be shed if you follow your program carefully. When you are not following your program your recording chart will tell the tale; use this information to stimulate your efforts to persevere.

The most valuable information you can obtain comes from your keeping a four-way chart.

Record your success in managing your behavior, the

amount you eat, the amount you exercise, and your weight—all on the same chart.

Make note of the days you meet the behavior-change objectives that you set for yourself, and each week indicate on your chart the number of days (0 through 7) that you have met these objectives. Keep track of the caloric value of the food you eat by using the calorie-equivalent exchange lists in the back of this book (these charts will be explained in Chapter 9); keep track of the caloric value of your exercise by using the charts provided for this purpose (to be explained in Chapter 10); and record your weight as measured on the same scale at the same time of the day *once each week* (daily weighing is *not* a good idea because weight fluctuates from one day to the next for many different reasons, and the information you get can be misleading).

Begin your graph in the same way as did the man whose results are shown in Figure 7 (Appendix D is a blank for your use). Take a "baseline" of how much you eat; exercise and weigh before you start your self-management program. (Note: Just counting the calories you eat will help reduce your food intake.) This will tell you where you are at the start and will help you evaluate your progress later. After about seven days of baseline, begin your "intervention" phase by making specific behavioral, eating, and activity plans. Keep the graph up to date faithfully and use it as the best guide possible to your personal planning. If you find that your weight is not changing even though your food intake is still low, increase your exercise. If you find you are losing weight more rapidly than two pounds weekly, you might be a little more generous with your food allowance. In other words, plan the management of your energy balance with the best possible outcome information at your disposal! Finally, if you find you are falling short of your behavior-change goals, answer these critical questions (page 82).

**Figure 7   Daily Eating, Exercise, and Weight Graph**

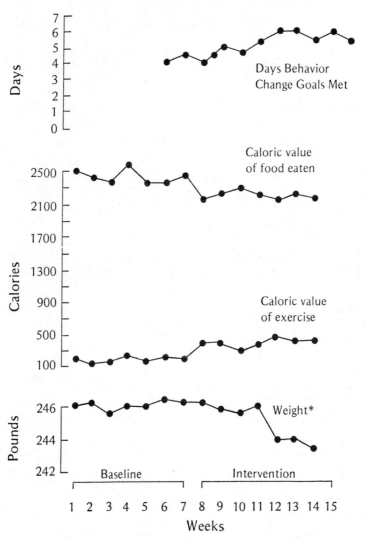

*Write in own weight range

1. Am I trying to do too much at one time?

2. Have I done all I can to cut down on my urge to eat so that my specific eating-control efforts can be successful?

3. Am I getting from others the help that I think I need and should have?

Depending upon the answers to these questions, you can work out a plan of attack to improve your long-range results.

In summary, you need payoff for your self-management efforts. Some of this payoff should come from relatives, friends, co-workers, or members of weight-control groups. You should also get some payoff from a graphic picture of your successes, a picture that, in the bargain, will help you toward even greater success.

In the next three chapters we will make suggestions for planning what you eat, for choosing a food plan, and how to use your body in a planned program of physical activity.

# Chapter 8
# Important Ideas in
# Planning What to Eat

In the first several chapters of this book we explained some sources of the urge to eat and suggested things you could do to bring these urges and your eating under control. In this chapter we will make some general suggestions about the choice of foods you eat; Chapter 9 will offer specific suggestions.

You have probably heard a great deal about a variety of different diets—the "low carbohydrate" diet, the "high fat" diet, the "grapefruit and cottage cheese" diet, even the "water" diet. It seems as though every month a new "diet discovery of a lifetime" appears in print in your local newspaper and promises miraculous weight losses with little effort on your part. You may have tried one or more of these diets only to find, as most people do, that you are too hungry or too weak to persevere for very long.

You don't want a diet that prescribes too little or too few of the foods you need to keep going. You do want a food plan that helps you select adequate amounts of all of the food you need for good nutrition and it should be a plan that you will be able to follow for life. That's a large order and that's what we would like to present to you now.

## WHY SHOULD YOU KNOW ABOUT NUTRITION?

Nutrition is the study of the essential chemicals in foods and the way they provide the body with energy and material for growth. These chemicals are called "nutrients" and there are approximately 50 nutrients (experts disagree about some, and others may be discovered), essentially proteins, carbohydrates, fats, vitamins, minerals, and water. We need all of these nutrients in the proper balance, and we suffer when we have too much or too little of these essential chemicals.

It is necessary to eat a variety of foods if we are to have all of the necessary nutrients. Many people believe that they will instinctively choose the right amounts of the proper foods, but this is not true. We receive signals from our bodies when they need food, but these signals tell us when, not what, to eat. Unfortunately, when we eat what we naturally choose to eat we tend to consume too much fat, too many sweets and foods with too much salt. Moreover, as large scale studies in both the United States and Canada have shown, our freely chosen diets may lack certain vitamins and minerals and may contain too many calories for our energy needs. These eating habits may affect our health, and diseases such as heart disease, hypertension, adult onset diabetes, and maybe even cancer may be influenced by what and how much we eat. *We need to choose our foods more wisely.*

With more than 10,000 items on the supermarket shelves, we have some difficult choices to make. With misinformation about nutrition being as common as a correct understanding of the facts, these choices are harder still. And with food packagers, advertisers, and marketers trying to guide our hands toward the more expensive foods, regardless of their nutritional values, wise selections are often more the exception than the rule. We turn to nutritional science to help us make these choices well.

## WHICH FOODS DO WE NEED?

To achieve the variety needed for health and satisfaction, people in most of the world's cultures have learned to choose their foods from among certain groups. Foods are generally grouped according to whether they are meats or other protein-rich foods, grains and cereals, milk and milk products (and other calcium-rich foods), and fruits and vegetables. Choosing foods from each of these groups is the means for devising a balanced food plan. Figure 8 (page 95) shows these basic food groups and the amounts of each recommended as a basis for good nutrition.

In different cultures different kinds of foods will be chosen from each group: The African Masai, for example, eat corn meal, a little meat, a mixture of blood and milk, and a variety of berries and leaves. The Asian vegetarian will choose wheat bread and rice, protein-rich lentils and legumes, cultured milk such as yogurt, and a variety of vegetables and tropical fruits. The Japanese, on the other hand, generally like rice, seafoods, some dairy products and calcium-rich bean curds, and many vegetables and seaweeds. Meanwhile, North Americans tend to prefer a fare of bread and rolls, beef, milk, potatoes, and salads and fruits. Each of these food preferences has been learned through years of cultural training. The people in one cultural tradition often frown on the food choices of others. But people in all cultures tend to have well-balanced diets when they can obtain a variety of the basic foods even though the nutrients are provided in different ways. Indeed, it is not unusual for the foods that are treasured in one culture to be viewed as waste in others.

In addition to choosing from each group of foods, it is also important to select a variety of foods within each group. This necessity stems from the fact that the foods in each group differ in their richness in varied nutrients. For example, meat is a good source of protein, B vitamins, and many minerals; but it is pork that is rich in vitamin B-1; liver and other organ meats that are high in iron; and fish that provides many of the nutrients of meat without the undesirable fat. Just as meats vary in their food values so, too, do vegetables and fruits. For example, dark-green leafy and yellow vegetables contain large amounts of vitamin A, while citrus fruits, melons, and berries contain more vitamin C than do other fruits. Therefore, just as it is important to build a food plan that includes some foods from each of the major groups, it is also important to choose a variety of foods within groups.

### SOME COMMON FOOD-PLAN ERRORS

We have found that people tend to make eight common errors in planning their food intake.

1. *Eating too much.* Chances are good that if you have read this far you eat too much. As we pointed out earlier, there is a proper amount of food for each person, an amount that provides just enough energy to keep you healthy and active. Whether we eat too much because we were inaugurated into the "clean platter club" as children, because we turn to food at times of stress, or because we just enjoy eating, we can pay a very high price for our indulgence.

In the next section we will offer some guidelines to help you determine how much food is enough, and how much is too much. Before we do, however, we would like to help you to understand some of the other common eating errors.

2. *Eating too much fat.* There is more concern and more misinformation about the role of fat in our diets than about any other nutrient. Therefore, we will spend a bit more time discussing fats than will be devoted to the other eating errors.

We need a certain amount of fat in our diet to preserve good health. Fat is necessary to help our bodies absorb certain vitamins like vitamins A, D, E and K. In addition, these vitamins are generally contained in the fat of foods. While our bodies can manufacture fat from proteins and carbohydrates, some of the fatty acids that we need cannot be made by the body and must be supplied by the food we eat. Fats are important building blocks in the trillions of cells in our bodies. They also assist in creating the chemical signals that tell us when to stop eating. As a final point they make food more palatable and help to reduce between meal hunger.

There are many different kinds of fats (more correctly called lipids by the chemists), but we will discuss the ones you are hearing about most frequently these days, namely saturates, cholesterol, polyunsaturates and mono-unsaturates.

Saturated fats make up 50% of butterfat, 48% of beef fat, 32% of chicken fat, and 40% of pork lard. Excessive quantities of saturated fat in our diets pose a problem because saturated fats tend to raise cholesterol levels in our bloodstreams, a process that is generally associated with atherosclerosis, or a clogging of the arteries, and these, in turn, may lead to stroke or heart attack.

It is important to understand some facts about cholesterol. It is also a lipid and it is both manufactured by the body from saturated fat and found in food as well. Cholesterol serves several necessary functions of the body but it can cause a problem as mentioned above when it collects in the arteries. Cholesterol is found in animal foods along with saturated fats. Therefore, since you are controlling the amount of saturated fat in your diet, you will be cutting down the amount of cholesterol that you consume at the same time.

Polyunsaturated fats in the diet may help to control the amounts of cholesterol in the blood and they are a source of the essential fatty acids (predominately linoleic acid) mentioned previously. Therefore, some should be included in the diet daily. Oils with polyunsaturates are also good sources of vitamin E. Most vegetable oils are rich in polyunsaturates (74% of safflower oil, 64% of sunflower oil, 58% of corn oil, 57% of soybean oil, and 51% of cottonseed oil). In contrast, animal fat is low in polyunsaturate content (3% of butter, 4% of beef tallow, 12% of pork lard, and 18% of chicken fat). Fish is a good food choice because it is low in total fat content and in addition fish fat is higher in polyunsaturates than other meats. It is also a good idea when buying margarine to check the label and choose brands with 35% or more poly-unsaturates and 18% or less saturates.

Mono-unsaturated fats are believed to be neutral with regard to their effect on the cholesterol in the blood. They are found in both animal and plant foods (72% of olive oil, 45% in chicken fat, and 42% of beef tallow).

It is important to reduce the level of total fat in your diet in order to reduce the caloric level of your intake. Because a tablespoon of fat has over twice as many calories as a tablespoon of sugar or starch (100 calories compared with 46 for sugar or starch), it is easy to see that many calories can be added to your intake if your diet is high in fat. Unfortunately, it is not always easy to spot the fat in our diets. For example, a T-bone steak has one-half as much fat as protein, while whole milk has as much fat as protein, and frankfurters have more fat than protein.

Important steps can be taken by reducing the amount of fat, especially saturated fat, that you eat. You can do this by using skim milk and skim milk products instead of whole milk, by choosing lean cuts of meat, substituting fish and fowl frequently for red meats, and by avoiding fried foods and fat-rich sauces and gravies. To include a source of poly-unsaturates in your diet, choose soft margarines and use vegetable oils with high polyunsaturate content when preparing food.

3. *Eating too much sugar.* There are at least three very good reasons for limiting the amount of refined sugars you eat. First, sugars provide energy but no other nutrients. Eating a large amount of sugar can therefore crowd many of the necessary nutrients out of your diet. Second, we tend to overeat sweets, ignoring the body's signal that enough new energy has been supplied. Indeed, when we turn to sugar for

an instant energy lift, we often experience a letdown a little later, leaving us less energetic than we would have been had we not eaten the treat. Finally, as is well known by now, sweet, sticky foods have a great influence upon tooth decay. In cultures where refined sugars are not included in the diet, people tend to have very strong, healthy, decay-free teeth.

While sweetness is an important taste that helps to keep our diets interesting, we can at least partially satisfy this desire by including fresh fruits in our diets.

4. *Eating too many "empty calorie" foods.* Sugars are one source of foods that have calories but no nutrients. Unenriched cereal products, many packaged snack foods, alcoholic beverages, and soft drinks are other sources. More and more of these foods are found in the marketplace where they are the subject of expensive promotional campaigns. They tend to be the most expensive calories you can buy, both in terms of dollars and in terms of their effect upon your general health. Virtually any amount of these foods is too much.

5. *Eating too much salt.* Primitive humans had very little salt in their diets, whereas in our modern culture we add a great deal of salt to our food. Such high salt diets are related to the development of hypertension (high blood pressure), especially in people prone to this condition. Therefore, it is important to moderate the amount of salt we eat. Trace amounts of salt occur in virtually all foods, and we consume sufficient salt in the normal course of eating to meet our bodily needs. When we choose foods with much extra salt added or when we add salt at the table, we generally move from sufficiency to excess. Thus it is wise to avoid these unnecessary and problematic sources of salt in selecting foods. This may take a little self-management, but the desire for saltiness in food is an *acquired* taste, not an *inbred* one, so we can train ourselves to enjoy less obviously salty foods.

6. *Eating too little fiber.* There has been growing recognition of the modern-day importance of another dietary element that was prevalent in the diets of our ancestors—fiber or roughage. This is nothing more than non-digestible bulk that is mostly found in whole grains and seeds, and in unprocessed fruits and vegetables.

It is estimated that Americans spend about $250 million yearly on laxatives which could largely be avoided by including more fiber in the diet. This fiber absorbs water from the large intestine and results in stools that are larger, softer and which promote good muscle tone and thus pass waste products regularly and rapidly out of our bodies. A lack of fiber in the diet has been associated with many of the health problems that are prevalent in modern industrialized societies such as diverticulitis, bowel cancer, heart disease, and obesity. You can increase the amount of fiber in your diet and, in addition, your supply of the trace nutrients that are lost when food is refined, by increasing your use of whole grain breads and cereals, by eating fruits and vegetables in their natural state, and by sometimes substituting dried peas, beans and nuts in place of meats.

7. *Eating too few fruits and vegetables.* As mentioned earlier, we consume about 40% fewer fresh fruits and 15% fewer fresh vegetables than we did some 40 years ago. Both are important elements in our diets for several reasons: They are good sources of essential nutrients; they are bulky, take more time to eat, and therefore give more eating satisfaction per calorie; and, as just mentioned, they are a very good natural source of fiber.

8. *Eating too few foods.* We tend to be creatures of habit. That means that we sink into ruts and do the same things repeatedly. We tend to eat certain familiar foods over and over again and do not experiment with new foods. Because only part of our satisfaction with food is its nutritional

value, when we eat a narrow range of foods we deprive ourselves of the stimulation associated with a variety of tastes, textures, and smells. We also minimize the likelihood that we will consume all of the needed nutrients, meaning that we will enjoy our eating less and get less benefit from it if we choose foods from lists that are too short. When we do this, we tend to eat too much in a vain effort to achieve the level of satisfaction that would be possible with lesser amounts of more varied food choices.

All of these mistakes are the results of bad decisions; all can be corrected by making decisions more wisely. While there is still some debate about certain of these considerations, there is wide agreement that your personal eating plan should contain:

1. The exact amount of energy you need.

2. No more than about 35% of its calories in fat, and as high a proportion of this fat as possible in polyunsaturate form.

3. A minimum of foods containing refined sugar and other "empty calorie" foods like soft drinks, alcoholic beverages, and snack foods.

4. A modest level of salt.

5. A reasonable amount of fiber.

6. A wide range of foods from the 4 food groups, including a large representation of fresh fruits and vegetables and whole grain and enriched cereal products.

Keeping these general guidelines in mind and consulting the labels on food packages can go far toward helping you plan your meals in a wise and healthful fashion.

## HOW MUCH SHOULD YOU EAT?

The amount of food you need depends on the energy you require. Your body needs energy to keep your heart pumping and your lungs breathing, to keep your body temperature up, your brain active, your muscles moving, and many other functions. This energy comes from either of two sources: It comes from the food you eat, or from the conversion of fat stored in the body into available energy. When you eat fewer calories than you need to keep going, you burn fat to provide this energy. When you eat more calories than you need, you store the excess as fat.

The National Academy of Sciences, through its National Council of Research, has worked out some Recommended Calorie Allowances for calories for the "average" man and woman of different ages. These recommendations will be found in Table 3. Use of these guidelines is not as easy as it seems, however, because there is no "average" person. People with bigger builds need more food energy to move their heavier bodies about; people who are more physically active also need more energy. People whose bodies use calories very efficiently need less energy than those whose bodies waste a good deal of the energy consumed. Therefore, the figures in this table are only starting points, and you will have to find the correct answer for yourself on a trial-and-error basis.

You will be better able to sustain weight loss if you plan to lose weight gradually. Rapid weight losses require a very great reduction in food intake and often leave you feeling constantly hungry and dissatisfied. You will not undergo this stress for long, and you will not learn habits sustainable for life when you use these unnatural methods. Therefore, you should plan a gradual reduction in food consumption which will lead to a gradual weight loss.

## Table 3  Daily Recommended Calorie Allowances

| Sex | Age | Weight (pounds) | Height (inches) | Energy (calories) |
|-----|-----|-----------------|-----------------|-------------------|
| Males | 11—14 | 97 | 63 | 2800 |
| | 15—18 | 134 | 69 | 3000 |
| | 19—22 | 147 | 69 | 3000 |
| | 23—50 | 154 | 69 | 2700 |
| | 51+ | 154 | 69 | 2400 |
| Females | 11—14 | 97 | 62 | 2400 |
| | 15—18 | 119 | 65 | 2100 |
| | 19—22 | 128 | 65 | 2100 |
| | 23—50 | 128 | 65 | 2000 |
| | 51+ | 128 | 65 | 1800 |
| Pregnant | | | | +300 |
| Lactating | | | | +500 |

Adapted from Food and Nutrition Board, National Academy of Sciences National Research Council Recommended Daily Dietary Allowances Revised 1974.

### ONE POUND PER WEEK IS AN IDEAL WEIGHT LOSS TARGET

Losing weight at this rate will allow you to learn new self-management skills while en route to your goal weight, and will give your body an opportunity to readjust internally to the new chemistry of a leaner you—both strong assets in your long-range efforts to control your weight.

To produce a one-pound loss per week, you must eat approximately 3500 fewer calories than you need to keep going; this means about 500 fewer calories per day. Consult Table 3 to find the recommended allowance for your sex and age, then reduce this number by 500 calories; this will be your starting level. Use it for two weeks and measure the effect upon your weight. If you have not lost weight, you can reduce your food intake a little more. However, keep these guidelines in mind:

**Women should eat at least 1200 calories per day unless under a doctor's supervision.**

**Men should eat at least 1500 calories per day unless under a doctor's supervision.**

If you eat at these levels and do not lose weight, you can plan increases in the amount of energy that you burn through activity. Suggestions will be made for this adjustment in Chapter 10.

It is a good idea to keep careful check on the level of your caloric intake and its effect upon your weight. Faithful use of the graph in Appendix D will give you a visual picture of this association. You will probably lose weight more rapidly at the start of your program because of fluid loss. You will experience plateaus in your weight loss because of changes in the level of salt in your body, changes in the level of your physical activity, and, of course, changes in the amount of food that you eat. Monitor these changes closely and adjust your food intake and energy expenditure levels appropriately so that you can keep up a weekly weight loss of approximately one pound. Then, when you have reached goal weight, you can continue this monitoring process so that you can keep your weight fluctuating within a natural two-to-four-pound range. (See Figure 7, page 81.)

Now that you have some guidelines for selecting foods and for determining how much to eat, we are ready to move into a discussion of exactly what you can eat to lose weight and how you can maintain your weight loss in a healthy way.

# Figure 8 Daily Food Guide

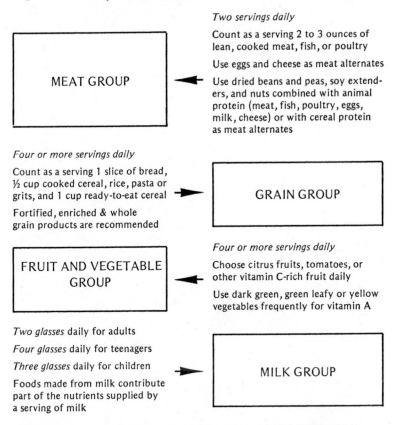

*Two servings daily*

Count as a serving 2 to 3 ounces of lean, cooked meat, fish, or poultry

Use eggs and cheese as meat alternates

Use dried beans and peas, soy extenders, and nuts combined with animal protein (meat, fish, poultry, eggs, milk, cheese) or with cereal protein as meat alternates

**MEAT GROUP**

*Four or more servings daily*

Count as a serving 1 slice of bread, ½ cup cooked cereal, rice, pasta or grits, and 1 cup ready-to-eat cereal

Fortified, enriched & whole grain products are recommended

**GRAIN GROUP**

**FRUIT AND VEGETABLE GROUP**

*Four or more servings daily*

Choose citrus fruits, tomatoes, or other vitamin C-rich fruit daily

Use dark green, green leafy or yellow vegetables frequently for vitamin A

*Two glasses* daily for adults

*Four glasses* daily for teenagers

*Three glasses* daily for children

Foods made from milk contribute part of the nutrients supplied by a serving of milk

**MILK GROUP**

CHOOSE A VARIETY OF FOODS FROM EACH GROUP EVERY DAY

95

# Chapter 9
# Choosing a Personal Food Plan Guide

Our food preferences are as individual as our finger-prints, but they are less stable because they change from time to time. Therefore, instead of asking you to follow a food plan that would appeal to the "average person," we would like to help you build your own plan by using a food-exchange system. This system has been developed by dieticians and physicians faced with the challenge of helping people plan their meals more wisely, but also allowing them to be guided in part by their individual tastes.

This system consists of five lists (called Exchange Lists) of foods: Grain, Meats and Meat Alternatives, Milk Products, Fruits and Vegetables, and "Miscellaneous" foods. You will find these in Appendix A at the back of the book. All of the foods in each list, *in the quantities specified*, are about the same number of calories. For example, in the grain list, 1/2 bagel, 3/4 cup of flake cereal, and 1/2 cup rice all have approximately 70 calories each. If your plan calls for one grain exchange, you could select any of the items on the list to meet this need.

It is important to bear in mind that everything you eat counts as an exchange on one of the lists. For example, if you select a slice of bread, you will have used one grain

97

exchange. If you butter the bread, that would be the use of one fat exchange from the miscellaneous list. Just about every food that you eat counts! The only foods that don't have to be counted are those listed as low-calorie extras. They may have a few calories, but the amounts are small so you may eat them in reasonable amounts without counting them as an exchange.

*UNDERSTANDING THE FOOD-EXCHANGE LISTS*
To help you understand the Food Exchange Lists, we would like to ask that you read through the Exchange Lists at the back of the book carefully (Appendix A); then read each of the following questions and write your answers directly in the space provided. You can verify your answers by checking on page 116. Be sure to read every question carefully and think about your answer, and about our answer if it is different from yours. To succeed in weight management, you must become an expert in your own food-related behavior, and learning these principles of good nutrition is an important tool.

1. Name the five Food Exchange Lists and give one example of the foods on each list. After the food, write the amount of that food allowed as one exchange:

| List | Food | Amount |
|------|------|--------|
| 1. *fat* | *butter* | |
| 2. *main* | *rice,* | *½ c. – 40 cals* |
| 3. *milk* | *skim* | *1 c. – 85 "* |
| 4. *meat* | | |
| 5. *veg.* | *beans* | |

Remember that all items on each list have the same

98

caloric value and can be exchanged with one another when caloric level is the basis of exchange. Remember, too, that the foods may differ in nutrient value; all of the foods are not exactly equal in their vitamin, mineral, and other nutrient content.

2. List the amounts of each of the following foods that can be eaten when the food plan calls for one meat exchange:

Chicken _____        Cottage cheese _____

Egg _____            Tuna fish _____

Peanut butter _____  Frankfurter _____

After you have worked with the lists for a while, you will learn how to quickly and accurately estimate the correct amount of each food item.

3. On which lists are the following foods found and how much is allowed for each exchange?

|                  | List | Amount |
| ---------------- | ---- | ------ |
| Corn on the cob  |      |        |
| Tomatoes         |      |        |
| Bacon            |      |        |
| Macaroni noodles |      |        |
| Broccoli         |      |        |
| Ice cream        |      |        |
| Kidney beans     |      |        |

As you use the lists for several days, you will learn food categories just as you will learn food quantities. Your initial challenge is to overcome some preconceived ideas about which foods belong where. For example, you may not have expected to find dried beans, peanut butter, and eggs all on the meats and meat alternative list, but each is a good source of protein.

4. Before you try to answer the next question, we would like to give you a tip: Most meat exchanges call for one ounce of meat, but an average serving of cooked meat may weigh three ounces and may therefore require three meat exchanges. It is also important to remember that while each meat exchange allows 75 calories, fatty meats, for example, are higher in calories than lean meats, so it is important to choose very lean meats and low-fat cheeses. Dried peas, beans, or lentils are other good choices because, when combined with a little animal protein or with a grain food, they give about the same food value as meat but without the fat. Choose those exchanges lower in fat whenever you can. It will be healthier for your arteries and better for your waistline. Now for the question:

If you have one ounce of cheese for breakfast, 1/2 cup tuna for lunch, and three ounces of chicken for dinner, how many meat exchanges will you have used for the day? _____

5. A tip will also help you correctly answer the next question: Each grain exchange supplies about 70 calories; the list includes a variety of breads and cereals plus some soups. Potatoes are also included as they are a starchy vegetable and are often used in place of a grain. Now the question:

If you choose 3/4 cup of cereal flakes for breakfast, a whole English muffin at lunch, and 1/2 cup serving of

rice for dinner, how many grain exchanges and how many calories will you have used in this way?
_____ exchanges _____ calories

6. If you choose 1 cup of skimmed milk for lunch and 3/4 cup skimmed-milk yogurt at dinner, how many milk exchanges will you have used? _____ Note that each milk exchange counts as 85 calories, assuming you use skimmed milk or partially skimmed milk. When you do buy skimmed milk, make certain it has been fortified with vitamins A and D. Notice also that cheese has been included on both the meat and the milk lists and is a good exchange on both lists. But when you eat it, count it as a serving of meat *or* milk, not both simultaneously.

7. Fruits and vegetables are found on the same list and each exchange supplies about 40 calories in the amounts stated. Notice that some fruits and vegetables on the list are better sources of vitamins than others and these are especially marked (in bold) on the list.

   Remember that many vegetables and some fruits are included as low-calorie extras and do not have to be counted as an exchange because they are very low in calories.

   How much of each of the following vegetables constitutes one exchange?

   carrots _____          tomato sauce _____

   tomato juice _____      corn _____

   beets _____            vegetable soup _____

   peas _____             spinach _____

   It's helpful to know that you can combine more than one vegetable to equal 1 exchange. If you had ½ tomato in your sandwich at lunch plus about ½ cup of carrots as carrot sticks, then that makes 1 exchange. Remember: If you add margarine to your vegetables you are using one fat exchange from the miscellaneous list.

8. What amount of each of the following fruits equals one fruit exchange?

| | |
|---|---|
| Apple juice | Applesauce |
| Orange | Raisins |
| Banana | Grapefruit |

Note that each of these fruits, in the amounts stated, have about 40 calories if they are eaten raw or cooked without sugar. If sugar is added or if the fruits are canned and sweetened, add miscellaneous exchanges for this sugar. Some fruits are better sources of vitamin C than others, and they are specially marked (in bold) on the exchange list.

9. A tip can help you to answer the next question: Certain desserts and beverages included in the miscellaneous list contain 80 calories in the amounts given. Don't forget to count these as *two* food exchanges, since the typical item on this list has about 40 calories. Now for the question:

> If you had 1 teaspoon of margarine, 1 tablespoon of French dressing, and 1/3 cup of ice cream today, how many miscellaneous exchanges would you have used?

———————

Remember the special problem posed by fats which are on the miscellaneous list. You should have some of the specially marked polyunsaturated fats in your food plan every day. Remember, too, to limit the empty calorie foods on this list as much as possible, and to be very careful to measure how much you eat of each, as it is very easy to lose track and eat too much before you realize what you are doing.

10. List the low-calorie extras that you enjoy eating. Realize that you can have reasonable amounts of these foods daily without counting them into your food plan. Many vegetables are included on this list, and we encourage you to eat them raw as snacks or salads. Some are common favorites when cooked as well. What are your favorite low-calorie extras?

_____    _____

_____    _____

_____    _____

11. Many people enjoy eating casseroles and mixed dishes. They can be used with this exchange system, but you must remember that each ingredient counts as one exchange. Now for the question.

Your daughter has prepared pizza for dinner, and you calculated that your portion consisted of 1 slice of bread, 1/4 cup tomato paste, and 2 ounces of low-fat cheese. List the type of exchanges you would have used and the number of each.

|  | Exchange | Number used |
|---|---|---|
| Slice of bread | _____ | _____ |
| 1/4 cup tomato paste | _____ | _____ |
| 2 ounces low-fat cheese | _____ | _____ |

12. Since evaluating these mixed dishes is a special challenge, we would like to give you one more chance to practice:

> Your mother-in-law has served spaghetti and meat balls. She knows you are trying to lose weight and has added no extra fat to the sauce. You eat 1/2 cup of spaghetti noodles, 1/2 cup of tomato sauce, and 2 meat balls that contain about 1 ounce of lean meat each. List the type of exchanges you have had and the number of each.

|  | Exchange | Number used |
|---|---|---|
| 1/2 cup spaghetti | _____ | _____ |
| 1/2 cup tomato sauce | _____ | _____ |
| 2 meat balls | _____ | _____ |

When you have answered these questions correctly, you have passed the first test: You know how to use the Food Exchange Lists properly. It will be important for you to remember to use the lists every day. When you are familiar with the lists, you will not have to check them for every item, but keep them handy so that you can look up new foods.

## CHOOSING THE PROPER PLAN

In the last chapter you learned how to calculate the number of calories you should have in your daily food plan. In Appendix B you will find several food plans, ranging from 1200 to 2300 calories per day. Each plan is within 20 calories of the number of calories specified. All are based on the Daily Food Guide found on page 95. Remember, women should eat at least 1200 calories and men 1500, unless under the supervision of a doctor. You will also recall that a reduction of 500 calories per day from the level that you need to keep going will generally produce a weight loss of about one pound per week.

Notice that each of the food plans contains a number of boxes. Each box represents one food exchange.

**Before you eat an item, write the current time of day in the box that corresponds to that item.**

Recording before you eat will help you to monitor food intake more accurately than will recording after the fact. Writing in the time of day will help you later in checking back to see if your eating is under the proper time control. Looking ahead at the empty boxes that remain for each day will give you an exact picture of how much of which foods you are still allowed, and this will help you in planning your eating wisely and well.

Figure 9 (page 106) offers an example of how one woman used the food plan. She used her milk exchange and fruit and vegetable exchanges as snacks, which is perfectly fine. Any extra foods eaten that are not in the daily allowance should still be recorded so that you can know exactly how many calories you are consuming. You will not lose weight because you think you are cutting down your caloric intake if, in fact, your extras bring your energy intake back up above your energy outflow. Record total calories in the space at the bottom of your food plan.

The food plans in this book have been developed for an adult with typical North American food habits. But your needs or tastes may differ somewhat from the average. You may be a teenager and need more milk than an adult, or you may prefer a diet with smaller amounts of animal protein and want more grain exchanges. Or you may just want to participate more actively in your food management program.

Work through the following steps and prepare your own personalized daily food plan.

## Figure 9 Daily Food Plan
### with Sample Recording of Intake

**1350–CALORIE FOOD PLAN**
EXCHANGES

| | 6 MEAT | 5 GRAIN | 2 MILK | 6 FRUIT & VEG | 4 MISC |
|---|---|---|---|---|---|
| **MORNING** | 8:00 | 8:00 | 10:30 | 10:30 | 8:00 |
| | | 8:00 | | | |
| **AFTERNOON** | 12:00 | 12:00 | 12:00 | 12:00 | 12:00 |
| | 12:00 | 12:00 | | 12:00 | 12:00 |
| **EVENING** | 6:00 | 6:00 | | 6:00 | 6:00 |
| | 6:00 | | | 6:00 | |
| | 6:00 | | | 9:00 | |
| **OTHER FOODS** | | | | | Extra margarine 40 calories |

| FOOD PLAN TOTAL 1350 | EXTRAS 40 | TOTAL CALORIES 1390 |
|---|---|---|

© Research Press Company

106

*STEP 1   THESE ARE YOUR
                MINIMUM REQUIREMENTS.*

Based on the Daily Food Guide (Figure 8) shown on page 95, an adult needs the minimum number of exchanges from our food exchange lists shown in the table below. Some days you will be eating vegetables as low-calorie extras and so you'll be getting more than your minimum needs for fruits and vegetables. This is a good habit to develop. It is also a good idea to include a source of fat or oil with polyunsaturates daily so we have added a miscellaneous exchange for that. Remember, children and teenagers need more milk exchanges than we have shown on the minimum requirement plan.

## MINIMUM REQUIREMENTS

| Exchanges | Meat | Grain | Milk | Fruit & Vegetable | Miscellaneous |
|---|---|---|---|---|---|
| Calories per exchange | 75 | 70 | 85 | 40 | 40 |

| | | | | |
|---|---|---|---|---|
| ☐ | ☐ | ☐ | ☐ | ☐ |
| ☐ | ☐ | ☐ | ☐ | |
| ☐ | ☐ | | ☐ | |
| ☐ | ☐ | | ☐ | |
| ☐ | | | | |

| Total calories per group | 375 | 280 | 170 | 160 | 40 |
|---|---|---|---|---|---|

Total calories on the minimum requirement plan = 1025

Don't be tempted to try this "minimum" as your diet. Remember our recommendation of no less than 1200 calories for a woman and 1500 calories for a man. By adding some additional exchanges to the minimum plan you will prevent those hunger pangs that result in loss of eating control and you will be adding a margin of nutritional safety to your food plan as well.

### STEP 2   HOW MANY CALORIES CAN I ADD TO THE MINIMUM PLAN TO LOSE 1 TO 1½ POUNDS A WEEK?

Let's use an example to show you how to calculate this. An average 15-year-old girl requires about 2100 calories a day (as shown in Table 3, page 93). To lose 1 pound a week, she has to be short 3500 calories a week or 500 calories a day.

$$\frac{3500 \text{ calories}}{7 \text{ (days)}} = 500 \text{ calorie deficit}$$

So on 1600 calories per day (2100−500=1600) she should lose a pound a week. She can therefore add 575 calories (1600−1025=575) worth of exchanges to the basic plan shown in Step 1.

Do *your* own calculations:

A.   Your normal daily caloric requirement as found in Table 3 _____

B.   Less 500 calories   − 500

C.   Less number of calories on basic plan   −1055

D.   Number of calories you can add to the basic plan (A−B−C) = _____

### STEP 3   HOW SHALL I SPEND THESE CALORIES ON EXTRA EXCHANGES?

Let's use our teenager again as an example. She has 575

calories a day to spend in extra exchanges.

| | |
|---|---:|
| She *needs* 2 more milk exchanges (2 x 85 calories) | 170 |
| She *wants* 1 more meat exchange (1 x 75 calories) | 75 |
| 2 more grain exchanges (2 x 70 calories) | 140 |
| 2 more fruit and vegetable exchanges (2 x 40) | 80 |
| 3 more miscellaneous exchanges (3 x 40 calories) | 120 |
| Total calories | 585 |

Don't worry if you are plus or minus 20 or so calories for your daily total.

How do *you* want to spend your extra calories?

Number of extra calories to spend = _____

| Number | Exchanges | Calories | |
|---|---|---|---|
| _____ | milk | ___ x 85 = | _____ |
| _____ | meat | ___ x 75 = | _____ |
| _____ | grain | ___ x 70 = | _____ |
| _____ | fruit & vegetable | ___ x 40 = | _____ |
| _____ | miscellaneous | ___ x 40 = | _____ |

Total extra calories = _____

### STEP 4 HOW SHALL I DISTRIBUTE MY TOTAL EXCHANGES THROUGHOUT THE DAY?

We strongly encourage you to have at least 3 meals a day. It's important for you to develop consistent, regular eating times. We will discuss the importance of this in the next section of this chapter. Figure 10 shows how our hypothetical teenager decided to distribute her exchanges. Notice that she likes to eat a snack when she comes home from school each day.

Use the blank Personalized Food Plan (Figure 11) on page 112 to develop *your* own food plan.

### WHEN YOU HAVE REACHED
### YOUR GOAL WEIGHT
Unless you are a very active person you are unlikely to lose weight with the more generous food plans that we have provided. However, once you have reached your goal weight and you wish to *maintain* that weight, you may find these plans very valuable indeed.

It is important to remember that weight maintenance is the result of *action carefully planned*, not of mere good luck. Therefore, you will have to always plan what you eat, using these recommendations as guides. To find the proper amount of food to eat, continue to graph what you eat, how much you exercise, and how much you weigh When your weight goes more than two to four pounds above goal you will know that it's time to cut down on what you eat and to increase your energy output.

### SOME SPECIAL POINTERS
Several hundred thousand people have now followed this food plan. We have learned much from their efforts and would like to pass their experiences along to you in the form of several pointers.

1. *Measure or weigh every food.* We all tend to make errors in estimating the quantities of the foods we eat—usually in the direction of underestimation. To correct this *natural* and *universal* distortion, it is important to measure or

## Figure 10  Personalized Food Plan

EXCHANGES

|  | 6<br>MEAT | 6<br>GRAIN | 4<br>MILK | 6<br>FRUIT & VEG | 4<br>MISC |
|---|---|---|---|---|---|
| **MORNING** |  | 8:00<br><br>8:00 | 8:00 | 8:00 |  |
| **AFTERNOON** | 12:00<br><br>12:00<br><br>4:00 | 12:00<br><br>12:00<br><br>4:00 | 12:00<br><br><br>4:00 | 12:00<br><br><br>4:00 | 12:00<br><br>12:00<br><br>4:00 |
| **EVENING** | 6:30<br><br>6:30<br><br>6:30 | 6:30 | 6:30 | 6:30<br><br>6:30<br><br>6:30 | 6:30 |
| **OTHER FOODS** |  |  |  |  |  |

| FOOD PLAN TOTAL | EXTRAS | TOTAL CALORIES |
|---|---|---|
|  |  |  |

111

## Figure 11 Blank Personalized Food Plan

### PERSONALIZED FOOD PLAN

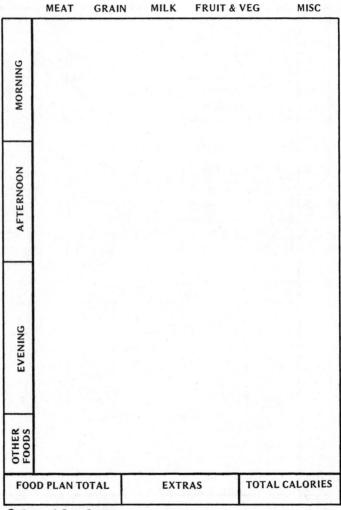

© Research Press Company

weigh every food you eat, at least for the first several weeks that you follow this program. Later you will become fairly accurate in your estimates, but from time to time you should go back to measuring and weighing just to keep your accuracy high. (See Appendix G, Equivalents by Volume.)

2. *Eat the foods at the time of day indicated.* There is some evidence that North Americans tend to pack most of their calories into one main meal, and this tendency may lead to an unnecessary build-up of fats in our bloodstreams and excess calories in fat storage. In addition, saving up most of our daily caloric allowance for one meal can lead to a condition of "semi-starvation" by day's end, with the result that far more is eaten at that large meal than is needed to keep us going. Following the general guidelines for the distribution of allowances throughout the day will help to guide you in a healthful meal distribution which, in the bargain, can be another aid in curbing your urge to overeat. Of course it is OK if you want to make small shifts such as using a fat exchange for margarine on your evening potato rather than on your bread at lunch. But do try to make these the exceptions and not the rule!

3. *Use nutrition labels whenever possible.* Labels tell you not only how much of certain nutrients the food contains, but also the caloric value of each serving. You know from your food plan that one meat exchange contains 75 calories. Look, for example, at the number of calories per serving on a can of chili con carne with beans. If 1 cup gives 330 calories, then 1/2 cup will give 165 calories, or approximately 2 meat exchanges. (Make it a scant 1/2 cup when serving yourself and check off 2 meat exchanges on your food plan.) You should also learn to use the labels to compare products before you buy them. Check the levels of fat, protein, and carbohydrates in different brands; check the percentage of your daily needs for the vitamins and minerals listed; and check to

see which product has the fewest calories per serving.

4. *Prepare your foods with great care.* Careless methods of food preparation can undo the potential benefit of very careful food selection. Therefore, you should take calorie-cutting steps whenever possible. Even the most famous French chefs are now experimenting with low-calorie cooking methods. Following are some suggestions to start you off on finding your own inventive ways.

a.  Choose lean meats and lean cuts of meat, removing all visible fat. Broil, boil, or bake in a manner that helps to melt the fat away. Throw out all fat that cooks out of the meat and cool all soups and stews long enough to be able to skim the fat that rises to the top. Cook poultry without the skin or remove the skin before eating it.

b.  Add flavor to your cooking with seasonings, herbs, bouillons, and fruit and vegetable juices. Cook fish with lemon juice and chopped onion; meats with fruit and vegetable juices and wines (the alcohol evaporates but the flavor stays!); and try cooking vegetables in bouillon or flavoring them with vinegar, lemon juice, or herbs. Make your own low-calorie salad dressing with tomato juice, herbs, and a little polyunsaturated oil.

c.  Use only low-calorie milk products in food preparation. For example, try yogurt and a little onion soup mix for salad dressings and vegetable dips. You can also use yogurt and green onions on potatoes, or spiced yogurt (i.e., yogurt with cinnamon) and fruit for dessert.

5. *Use special low-calorie preparations sparingly, if at all.* You are conditioning yourself to permanent eating habits that you will follow for the rest of your life. Therefore, it is not a good idea to build up a dependency on artificially sweetened foods. These *may* even be harmful to your health if eaten in large quantities over long periods of time. So use them as sparingly as possible and read the food label to be sure that the food is in fact low in calories. Remember that "low-cal" is *not* "no-cal," so you must read the label to determine the number of calories per serving and count these items as an exchange or part of an exchange in your daily allowances.

Now you know why you should eat certain foods, how much you should eat, and how to keep track of the amount of your food intake and behavioral self-management success as they bear upon your weight loss. You are three-fourths of the way home and have one lap left to go: learning how to build physical activity into your day so that you can work your appetite down, elevate your spirits, condition your body, and burn extra energy to speed your loss of weight. Physical activity is the topic of the following chapter.

Answers to questions on the use of the exchange lists.

| | List | Food | Amount |
|---|---|---|---|
| 1. | Meat | Your own example | Check exchange lists |
| | Grain | " | " |
| | Milk | " | " |
| | Fruit and vegetables | " | " |
| | Miscellaneous | " | " |

2. 1 ounce chicken
1 egg
1 tablespoon peanut butter
1/3 cup cottage cheese
1/4 cup tuna
1 small frankfurter

| | | List | Amount |
|---|---|---|---|
| 3. | Corn on the cob | Fruit and Vegetable list | 1/2 medium ear or 1/3 cup |
| | Tomatoes | Fruit and Vegetable list | 1 large or 1 cup |
| | Bacon | Miscellaneous list | 1 slice |
| | Macaroni noodles | Grain list | 1/2 cup |
| | Broccoli | Fruit & Vegetable list | 1 cup |
| | Ice cream | Miscellaneous list | 1/3 cup |
| | Kidney beans | Meat list | 1/2 cup |

4. Number of exchanges = 6

5. Number of exchanges = 4    Number of calories = 280

6. Number of exchanges = 2

| 7. | Carrots | 1 cup | Tomato sauce | 1/2 cup |
| | Tomato juice | 1 cup | Corn | 1/2 medium or 1/3 cup |
| | Beets | 3/4 cup | Vegetable soup | 1/2 cup |
| | Peas | 1/2 cup | Spinach | 1 cup |
| 8. | Apple juice | 1/2 cup | Applesauce | 1/2 cup |
| | Orange | 1 small | Raisins | 1 1/2 tablespoons |
| | Banana | 1/2 | Grapefruit | 1/2 |

9. Number of exchanges = 4

10. Your choice

11. 1 grain exchange
1 fruit and vegetable exchange
2 meat exchanges

12. 1 grain exchange
1 fruit and vegetable exchange
2 meat exchanges

# Chapter 10
# **Exercise**

Now that you have learned about situational and nutritional control, it is time to go on to the most forgotten element in weight control: the proper use of exercise.

*WHAT IS EXERCISE,*
*WHY IS IT NEEDED,*
*AND WHO NEEDS IT?*

Exercise is any action which makes the body muscles work, such as walking, running, pushing, pulling, throwing, lifting, and climbing. The body needs exercise for health and well-being, and the lack of exercise can lead to serious problems. For example, muscle and joint diseases, heart disease, and obesity are more likely to occur among inactive people. Research has shown that obese people are far less active than nonobese people, and that inactivity makes it very difficult for the obese person to use up, as energy, all the calories he eats.

Until now people did not take the role of exercise seriously for three reasons. First, it was believed that a very large amount of exercise would be needed to burn up enough calories to do any good. For example, it has been said that you would have to climb up and down the stairs of the

Empire State Building for 4 hours, or chop wood for 7 hours, or walk for 14 hours in order to use up 1 pound of body fat. If your goal were to lose a great many pounds in a short time, you would be hard pressed to reach it through this type of exercise. But if you were smarter about weight loss and knew that weight lost is too often weight quickly regained, then these numbers would have a different meaning for you. You would realize that fairly fast walking for one hour per day (for example, to and from the store or to work) could add up to the loss of one pound within two weeks—25 pounds within a year.

A second incorrect idea people have about exercise is the belief that exercise causes an increase in hunger when, in fact, the opposite seems to be true. Our bodies have their own signal systems that tell us when to start and stop eating; but for some reason that scientists do not yet understand, these signals work well only in the bodies of active people. Studies of rats have shown that when they were not allowed to exercise, they ate and grew fat, but when exercise was allowed, the rats ate less and remained at normal weight. Farmers have learned this trick too: When they want their animals fat for market, they keep them penned up. People who are penned up go through the same fattening process—the less they do, the more they eat. Naturally, if they start to do very active things like hard physical labor all day long, they will eat more, but if they increase their activity *just a little*, they will usually eat less. As a side benefit, a little exercise will also make people less likely to become bored, less physically and mentally tired; and these, too, are important gains. Exercise can also help rid you of tension and anger. Next time you are bored, tired, tense, or angry, try going for a fast walk for a few minutes and note the changes in the way you feel.

A third incorrect idea people have about exercise is that it is modern to avoid exercise. It is true that we live in a world that spends billions of dollars every year to avoid exercise. We try to save exercise in the ways we move from place to place: The long walk gave way to the bicycle, the bus, and now the car; the trek from a parking place to a store has given way to parking-lot-at-the-door shopping centers; stairs have been replaced by escalators and elevators to make certain we use as little energy as possible. In industry, machines are doing most of the hard work, which is good in several ways (there are probably fewer accidents and women are better able to work along with men because huge muscles are no longer needed), but bad in others because jobs require less effort (and thus fewer calories) and are less interesting. Our homes are equipped so as to minimize our energy output: Machines such as the electric vacuum cleaner, dishwasher, clothes washer and dryer, and mixer help us with our housework; ice cream freezers, ice crushers, and can openers are all electric; and all these gadgets work against women who are concerned with watching their weight. In his workshop or out in the garden, the man of the house is no better off. He uses an electric drill and saw instead of a brace and bit and handsaw; gasoline or electric lawn mowers and hedge cutters are used instead of human-powered tools. All of these gadgets take away chances for useful exercise, and people actually feel deprived if they don't own machines of this sort. While this may be good for industry, it is surely a problem for the individual.

So far we have described what exercise is and why it is needed. We have not yet, however, talked about who needs it. Everyone physically able to move needs exercise; even people who cannot get out of bed must use whatever muscles they can. All people need exercise, both to maintain good health and to avoid obesity. Dr. Jean Mayer said: "If we want to avoid obesity, we must either exercise more or feel hungry all our lives." People who are already overweight have an even greater need to exercise to ensure weight loss and to assist an already overburdened heart and blood-supply system.

## WHAT KIND OF EXERCISE DO YOU NEED?

Because people are beginning to accept the fact that exercise is important, exercise fads are developing much like the food fads that have been popular in recent years. Like the food fads, most of the exercise fads are useless. They promise to "roll away fat," "restore your youthful figure," and "build muscles like iron," all in two to four weeks with no effort on your part. This is, of course, as silly as saying that you can lose twenty pounds in two weeks without even trying.

There are many different kinds of exercise, but for our purposes we need speak only of three  The first is called "passive" exercise because you are asked to do nothing more than keep pace with some electric or mechanical gadget. However, the gadget supplies its own power, and you get little good from using it. You may move your limbs a little, but you will neither work muscles nor use many calories. The second is called "isometric" exercise. In these exercises you pit muscles against one another or against a fixed object such as a door frame. These exercises do build muscle strength, but because they are done for very short periods of time and exercise only a very few muscles, they burn very few calories.

Activities that are the most healthful and expend the most calories are dynamic exercises that require the use of large amounts of muscle and involve moving the body through distance. These types of exercises may be of moderate intensity, such as bowling, golf, and walking leisurely. When carried on for longer periods of time and done regularly, they use up calories and are a health benefit. However, because of the time involved they often tend to be done only once in a while. Dynamic exercises that are strong enough and last long enough to make your heart beat faster, that make you huff and puff and sweat a little, are often called "aerobic" exercises. They include such activities as walking briskly, jogging, cycling, and swimming, and they involve moving large amounts of muscle mass through distance. When done regularly, these types of exercise will build up the strength of your heart and burn up a goodly number of calories.

### HOW MUCH EXERCISE DO YOU NEED?

Begin exercising gently and increase gradually. Sudden, very difficult exertion may be harmful, and too much of anything is bad. You will have to find your own level, a level that will help you to reach your goals of fitness and weight loss. In general, we feel people should try to *build up* to the use of an *extra* 500 calories per day through exercise. Notice that the key word here is *extra*. If you are to benefit from your exercise, it must be in addition to the energy which you already spend in going about your daily business.

We like to think of exercises as falling into three groups: light, moderate, and heavy. As you can see in Table 4 (page 124), light exercise burns four calories per minute, moderate exercise burns seven calories per minute, and heavy exercise burns ten calories per minute (see also Appendix F for a more detailed list). These calorie values are not true for everyone at all times because people doing each of these things will do them a little differently and will thus use more or less energy. Also, they include the amount of energy you would use if you were lying quietly at rest; but they are good averages. By working with these averages you can decide whether you want to exercise lightly for a longer time one day or heavily for a shorter time the next so as to reach your goal for energy use for the day.

To figure out how much exercise you should do, follow the same steps you used in figuring out how many calories you should eat. First, use the chart in Figure 12 (page 126) as a model (a blank is included at the back of this book in Appendix C) to record how often you do each of the listed items in the normal course of your day. This will give you the baseline of your activity. It is very important that you "tell it like it is." Do not do more or less than you usually do when

123

#### Table 4  Average Energy Expenditure During Recreational Activities*

| Light Exercise 4 calories/minute | Moderate Exercise 7 calories/minute | Heavy Exercise 10 calories/minute |
|---|---|---|
| Dancing (slow step) | Badminton (singles) | Calisthenics (vigorous) |
| Gardening (light) | Cycling (9.5 mi./hr.) | Climbing stairs (up & down) |
| Golf | Dancing (fast step) | Cycling (12 mi./hr.) |
| Table tennis | Gardening (heavy) | Handball, paddleball, squash |
| Volleyball | Stationary cycling (moderately) | Jogging |
| | | Skipping rope |
| Walking (3 mi./hr.) | Swimming (30 yd./min.) | Stationary cycling (quickly) |
| | Tennis (singles) | Stationary jogging |
| | Walking (4.5 mi./hr.) | Swimming (40 yd./min.) |

*Values are for gross energy expenditure

you figure out your baseline. Decide which kind of exercise you will want to choose—for example, walking, or some sport or physical work—and then decide whether you want to be lightly, moderately, or heavily active. Then plan how many minutes you would like to do each of these exercises each day. We suggest that you try to build up slowly:

| First Week: | Use 59 to 150 extra calories |
| Second Week: | Use 100 to 250 extra calories |
| Third Week: | Use 150 to 350 extra calories |

| Fourth Week: | Use 200 to 500 extra calories |
| Fifth Week: | Use 250 to 500 extra calories |

If you exercise this way, you will not strain yourself and you will be more comfortable with your program. We think 250 calories per week (that would mean walking at a slow pace for about one hour) should be your minimum for the first five weeks; but it is important never to fall below this level once you have begun.

Because it is not easy to figure out the caloric value of exercise, we would like to give you some practice. (Refer to Figure 12 for assistance.) Try to solve the following problem: During the weekdays you have decided to start an exercise program consisting of two 20-minute walks per day (3 miles per hour) instead of your normal coffee breaks, and you have decided to climb the stairs to your office instead of using the elevator so that you will spend 5 extra minutes per day climbing stairs. As you become more fit, you also decide to jog in place for 7 minutes each weekday as you watch the evening news on TV, and you increase this 7-minute exercise to 3 times each weekend day.

1. How many calories will you use up each week on this plan?

2. How many pounds will you lose following this plan for a week?

3. How many pounds will you lose if you follow this plan for one year?

*Answers*

1. Walking 3 miles per hour uses 4 calories per minute; walking 20 minutes thus uses 80 calories; doing this twice each day uses 160 calories; and doing it five

## Figure 12  Exercise Plan*

Light exercise — Each box = 5 min. = 20 calories

Dancing (slow step)
Gardening (light)
Golf
Table tennis
Volleyball
Walking (3 mi./hr.)

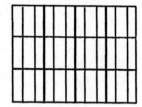

___ x 20 = _____

Moderate exercise — Each box = 5 min. = 35 calories

Badminton (singles)
Cycling (9.5 mi./hr.)
Dancing (fast step)
Gardening (heavy)
Swimming (30 yd./min.)
Tennis (singles)
Walking (4.5 mi./hr.)

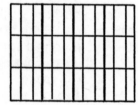

___ x 35 = _____

Heavy exercise — Each box = 5 min. = 50 calories

Calisthenics (vigorous)
Climbing stairs (up & down)
Cycling (12 mi./hr.)
Handball, paddle ball, squash
Jogging
Skipping rope
Stationary cycling (quickly)
Stationary jogging
Swimming (40 yd./min.)

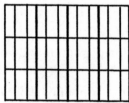

___ x 50 = _____

*Caloric values are for gross energy expenditure    Daily Total _____ times each week uses 800 calories. Climbing stairs uses 10 calories per minute; climbing stairs for 5 minutes per day uses 50 calories; doing this five times per week uses 250 calories. Jogging in place also uses 10 calories per minute; jogging for 7 minutes uses 70 calories, which would result in the use of 350 calories during weekdays; jogging 3 times for 7 minutes each weekend day uses 420 calories, making a total use of 770 calories through jogging. Therefore, you will use 800+250+770 calories per week, or 1820 calories.

2.  You can expect to lose 1/2 pound each week because 1820 is a little more than one half of 3500 (the number of calories needed to get rid of one pound of fat).

3.  At this rate you will lose 26 pounds within one year (52 x 1/2 pound).

## WHAT CAN YOU DO
## TO BE SURE TO KEEP EXERCISING?

This is a very important question. Dr. Donald Smith of the University of Michigan has described what he calls the "four-day phenomenon"—people who start out to do things for their own good are not likely to keep doing them for more than four days. Nobody knows what magic there is in four days but diets, exercise programs, New Year's resolutions and many other good intentions seem to last for four days and no more. We have found that there are a few things which you can do to make it more likely that you will follow through on an exercise program.

### First, find a partner

If you have a partner to exercise with, you can make it a social experience which will be more fun. Also, if you have a partner who expects to exercise, and his exercise depends upon you, you will keep up your end so that he keeps up his.

### Second, choose wisely

Pick an exercise which suits your style of living and your place of living. If you are not sports-minded or if you are embarrassed to exercise in public, you will do best to choose walking, gardening, climbing stairs, or the like. If you like to compete and don't mind an audience, a sport might be your cup of tea. Also, a wise exercise choice is one that you can do throughout the year. For example, if you live in a warm area, skiing is not likely to be something you can do all year round.

### Third, exercise naturally

When people depend upon unusual activities for all of their exercise, they are less likely to follow through than if they make exercise a natural part of the day. Therefore, plan to walk to work or to the store, and if it takes too long, jog part of the way to speed things up. Find as many ways as you can to build exercise into the natural course of your day, like standing instead of sitting to iron, walking around while waiting for a friend, and always using stairs instead of elevators.

### Fourth, pay yourself off

By choosing an exercise you enjoy, you give yourself some payoff for your efforts. Find other payoffs: if the scenery bores you, carry a transistor radio when you walk; graph your exercise; show the graph to people who count and let them praise you. Or pay yourself off in other ways. For example, in one family the husband takes out the garbage if the wife makes five trips up and down the stairs. If you will do these four things—exercise with a partner, choose your exercise carefully, build it into the natural course of your day, and make sure that there is a payoff—you are likely to be able to get over the four-day limit and set yourself on a course. Believe it or not, once you begin to get yourself on some sort of regular exercise program, you will miss it on days when you do not follow through and you will feel much more alive and well on days when you do.

# Chapter 11
# **Your New Beginning**

You have worked hard to reach this point. You have learned that there are many physiological, social, and psychological advantages associated with weight control. You have also learned that your weight is under the influence of many different forces, some biological, some psychological, and many social and situational. Therefore, management of weight in our "fat world" requires mastery of living situations rather than being the crisis of "will power" that you may have believed it to be. To make this situational control possible, we have analyzed eating as the result of an urge and have shown that you have many choicepoints at which you can act to weaken your urge to eat. We have suggested that your urge to eat is more likely to be psychologically than physiologically motivated, and that control of this urge often requires important and lasting changes in your general style of living. We urged you to select a personal program of action, starting with any of several steps that are antecedents to eating, followed by eating itself, and, finally, the consequences of eating. For review, we offer the following list of these techniques.

## ANTECEDENTS
*Put you in the picture --*

A–1 Keep a record of the conditions under which you eat

A–2 Manage your eating-related feelings by:

1. Controlling hunger through eating three well-balanced, planned meals.

2. Controlling fatigue by making certain that you have an adequate amount of sleep nightly.

3. Controlling boredom by planning to include new and stimulating activities into your daily schedule.

4. Controlling unhappiness by setting reasonable and achievable expectations about how much enjoyment your daily activities will bring and by working to improve the quality of your daily life.

5. Controlling anger by expressing your desires to others in order to structure situations in the most positive way possible.

6. Controlling tension by planning rest breaks and learning to relax through meditation.

7. Coping with happiness by learning to reward yourself with things, other than treats, as a celebration.

8. Coping with problem moods when they do occur by turning to nonfood activities, engaging in physical activity or, if need be, choosing a small amount of a non-preferred food.

A–3 Thinking your way to constructive action by thinking through the expected events of the day and imaging yourself acting in the most positive *possible ways and planning means through which you will translate obstacles into opportunities.*

*A—4   Controlling the availability of problem foods by:*

1. Resisting the urge to buy the wrong foods by shopping from a list, only after a full meal, and by avoiding exposure to displays of foods that you should not eat.

2. Having nonproblem foods on hand, having problem foods on hand only if they require considerable effort in preparation, and keeping these and all foods stored in covered containers in the kitchen only.

*A—5   Retraining your urge to eat by:*

1. Making eating a "pure" experience by engaging in no problem activities other than socializing with your family while you eat.

2. Eating only in the kitchen or dining room and there only when sitting down at your personal place.

3. Planning specific times of day for all meals and snacks.

*EATING BEHAVIORS PER SE*

*B—1   Record what you plan to eat before you eat*

*B—2   Control the amount that you eat by:*

1. Pausing for two to five minutes before beginning to eat at mealtimes.

2. Slowing the rate of eating by placing utensils on your plate after every mouthful and not picking them up again until after the food has been swallowed.

3. Waiting 10 minutes before beginning to eat any un-planned snack.

*B—3  Control the size of the portion that you take by:*

1. Measuring every helping.

2. Making normal portions appear to be as large as possible.

3. Making second helpings difficult to get.

## MANAGING THE CONSEQUENCES OF EATING

*C—1  Build social support for your successful actions by:*

1. Identifying the people who are most likely to be of help to you—relatives, friends, or a weight-control group.

2. Informing them of your plans.

3. Asking for their positive response to your positive actions.

*C—2  Record your success in behavior change, eating and activity patterns, and weight change*

Think through each of these recommendations and attempt to convince yourself of their rationale and value. If you have difficulty doing this, refer back to the point in this book at which each technique was introduced and read slowly through its discussion. If you feel the need for further clarification, read the discussion of the technique in our longer book *Slim Chance in a Fat World* (Professional Edition) or in Dr. Stuart's book *Act Thin: Stay Thin.* (Both of these books can be ordered from Research Press Co., 2612 N. Mattis Ave.,

Champaign, IL 61820).

When you have your life situation and your behavior under better control, we suggest that you undertake a plan to control what you eat and how you expend energy. We urge you to:

1. Set a weight-loss goal of 1 to 2 pounds per week.

2. Cut your food intake somewhat, but also increase your energy expenditure to some degree.

3. Eat at least 1500 calories daily if you are a man and 1200 calories daily if you are a woman.

When you have figured your calorie limit, ask yourself several important questions about what you eat:

1. Are you eating too much food?

2. Are you eating too much fat?

3. Are you eating too much sugar?

4. Are you eating too many empty calories?

5. Are you eating too many highly processed foods?

6. Are you eating too few fruits and vegetables?

7. Are you eating enough different foods?

Once you have found answers to some of these questions, select the proper program for yourself, ranging from 1200 to 2300 calories. To pick the right plan, find out your basic daily calorie needs and subtract 500 calories to give you a one-pound-per-week weight loss.

As you start to get your eating under control, begin to attend to the way you exercise. Exercise will not only help you lose weight and control tension, but it can also do a world of good for your heart. To see how much exercise you need, begin by taking an exercise "baseline" as you did an eating baseline. From this baseline add at least 250 calories worth of exercise per day and then decide how you want to do it—through light, moderate, or heavy walking, sports, or work. Then take a few steps to make sure that you will beat the "four-day phenomenon":

1. Find a partner, seek professional help, or join a weight-control group.

2. Choose your exercise wisely.

3. Build exercise into the natural course of your day.

4. Give yourself a payoff.

You can use exercise in at least two ways. If you want to eat a little more, you can exercise a little more; and if you know that you will be overeating at a party, do some extra exercise *in advance.*

Perhaps the most important thing to say in closing is that to lose weight you will have to make important changes in the way you go about living. You will have to make sure that the situation in which you live makes the right kind of eating easy. You will have to be smart in choosing what you eat, when you eat, where you eat, and how you prepare what you eat. And you will have to be as active as you possibly can both to make weight loss easier and to make life longer and fuller. Whenever you come to a problem—and there will be many—consider it as a challenge. Solve the problem—do not submit to it. If you solve it, you can go on and free yourself from the pain of obesity. If you submit, you will be dooming yourself to continued suffering. What you must change, in a word, is not only what you eat and what you do, but also how bold you are in the way you go about changing.

# Appendix A
# **Food Exchange Lists**

All foods within each exchange list, in the amounts specified, are approximately equal in caloric content. It is essential that foods be weighed or measured until such time as portions can be estimated accurately.

## LOW-CALORIE EXTRAS
(Negligible calories)

The following foods, seasonings, and beverages are very low in calories. They may be eaten freely in reasonable amounts and do not have to be recorded on the daily food plan.

Bouillon, broth
Carbonated beverages (sugar free)
Coffee, tea
Herbs, spices, onion flakes
Gelatin, rennet tablets
Pickles (unsweetened)
Mustard, soy sauce, vinegar, garlic, horseradish
Artificial sweetener

Fruits (unsweetened): cranberries, rhubarb, lime juice, lemon juice
Vegetables (cooked or raw): asparagus, beans (young-green, yellow), bean sprouts, cabbage, cauliflower, celery, chives, cucumber, endive, lettuce, mushrooms, peppers, radishes, sauerkraut, summer squash, watercress, zucchini squash

Pages 143-151 can be duplicated without written consent from the publisher.

# MEATS AND MEAT ALTERNATIVE EXCHANGE LIST
(75 calories per exchange)

Each meat exchange supplies approximately 75 calories of energy. Those on List 1 are lower in fat and will generally average somewhat less than this amount and those on List 2 are higher in fat and will average somewhat more. An average serving of cooked meat weighs approximately 3 ounces, which would be 3 meat exchanges. It is recommended that 2 servings of meat or meat alternates, weighing 2 to 3 ounces each, be eaten daily.

**List 1.** The following are *lean* meats, *low-fat* cheeses and high protein vegetables. Make at least half your meat choices from this list.

Meat and poultry

| | | Cheese | |
|---|---|---|---|
| Chicken, game meats, liver and other organ meats, pheasant, rabbit, turkey, veal | 1 ounce | Cottage cheese | 1/3 cup |
| | | Skimmed or partially skimmed milk | 1 1-inch cube or 1 ounce |
| Fish | | High Protein Vegetables | |
| Bass, cod, flounder, haddock, halibut, lobster, salmon, trout, etc. | 1 ounce | Baked beans in sauce (no pork) | 1/4 cup |
| Crab, lobster, salmon, tuna (water pack) | 1/4 cup (loosely packed) | Dried beans, peas, lentils (cooked whole or soup) | 1/2 cup |
| Clams, oysters, scallops, shrimp | 3-5 medium | | |

**List 2.** The following meat exchanges contain *more fat;* these should be used more sparingly.

Meat and poultry

| | | | |
|---|---|---|---|
| Beef, duck, goose, ham, lamb, pork | 1 ounce | Peanut butter | 1 tablespoon |
| Eggs | 1 egg | Cold cuts - bologna, salami, etc. | 1 slice (4 1/4 x 4 1/4 x 1/8-inches) |
| Cheese | | | |
| American (processed), cheddar, Edam, Swiss, etc. | 1 slice (4 x 4 x 1/8-inches) or 1 1-inch cube or 1 ounce | Frankfurters (12 per lb.) | 1 small |
| | | Sausage | 1 small link |

# GRAIN EXCHANGE LIST
## (70 calories per exchange)

Each grain exchange supplies approximately 70 calories of energy. Some soups and potatoes have been included on the Grain Exchange List. At least three servings of whole grain or enriched breads or cereals should be eaten daily.

Breads and rolls
 Bread, white, whole-wheat, 1 slice
   rye
 Bread dressing, or stuffing   2 tablespoons
 Hamburger, hot dog bun        1/2 bun
   (large)
 Matzos                        1 6-inch diameter
 Melba toast, thin             5 slices
Quick breads
 Biscuit, roll, muffin         1 2-inch diameter
 Corn bread                    1 piece 1 1/2-inch cube
 Doughnut, plain               1 small
 English muffin                1/2
 Pancake                       1 4-inch diameter
                               cake
 Tortilla                      1 6-inch diameter
                               tortilla
 Waffle                        1 4-inch diameter
                               waffle

Crackers
 Graham                        2 crackers, 2 1/4-
                               inches square
 Oyster                        1/2 cup
 Round                         5 crackers, 2-inches
                               diameter

Rye
 Saltines                      2 double crackers
                               5 crackers, 2-
                               inches square
 Soda                          3 crackers, 2 1/2-
                               inches square
Cereals
 Cooked: grits, oats, rice,    1/2 cup
   wheat, barley
 Ready-to-eat: flake and       3/4 cup
   puff types
 Wheat Bran (natural)          1/2 cup
 Wheat Germ                    2 rounded
                               tablespoons
 Popcorn (no added fat)        1 1/2 cups
Pastas (cooked, noodles only)
 Egg noodles, macaroni,        1/2 cup
   spaghetti
Potatoes                       1 medium or
                               1/2 cup

Soups
 Soup: barley, noodle, rice    1 cup
 Soup: cream (made with        1/2 cup
   water)

# MILK EXCHANGE LIST
## (85 calories per exchange)

Each milk exchange supplies approximately 85 calories of energy. Skimmed or partially skimmed milk should be used. Two cups of milk or its equivalent should be drunk daily. Children should have 3 cups and teenagers 4 cups daily.

| | | | |
|---|---|---|---|
| Buttermilk (skimmed) | 1 cup (8 ounces) | Evaporated milk | 1/4 cup |
| Cheese, American processed, cheddar, edam, etc. (use skimmed or partially skimmed milk cheese more frequently) | 1 ounce, 1 inch cube, or 1 slice | Evaporated milk (skimmed) | 1/2 cup |
| | | Nonfat dried milk powder | 1/3 cup |
| | | Partially skimmed milk | 3/4 cup |
| | | Skimmed milk | 1 cup |
| | | Yogurt, plain | 1/2 cup |
| | | Yogurt, plain (made from skimmed milk) | 3/4 cup |

# FRUIT AND VEGETABLE EXCHANGE LIST
## (40 calories per exchange)

Each fruit and vegetable exchange, in the amount specified, supplies approximately 40 calories of energy.

Fruits may be fresh, dried, cooked, canned, or frozen as long as *no sugar* is added. Those in bold type are especially rich in vitamin C. At least two exchanges of fruit should be eaten daily, with one being rich in vitamin C.

Vegetables may be eaten either raw or cooked and two or more vegetables may be combined to equal 1 exchange. At least 2 exchanges of vegetables should be eaten daily. Those in bold type are especially rich in vitamins; choose them frequently.

| | | | |
|---|---|---|---|
| Apple, guava, nectarine, orange, peach, pear | 1 small | Strawberries, cantaloupe, honeydew melon, watermelon | 1 cup |
| Banana, grapefruit, mango, papaya | 1/2 | Cherries, grapes | 12 |
| | | Raisins | 1 1/2 tablespoons |
| Apricots, figs, plums, prunes | 2 | Juice: apple, grapefruit, orange, pineapple | 1/2 cup |
| Applesauce, pineapple, blackberries, blueberries, raspberries | 1/2 cup | Juice: grape, prune | 1/4 cup |

| | | | |
|---|---|---|---|
| Bamboo shoots, broccoli, carrots, eggplant, greens (beet greens, chard, collards, dandelion, kale, mustard greens, spinach, turnip greens), kohlrabi, okra, turnip | 1 cup | Artichokes, beets, Brussels sprouts, leeks, onions, okra, pea pods | 3/4 cup |
| | | Peas, pumpkin, rutabagas, winter squash, water chestnuts | 1/2 cup |
| | | Corn, parsnips | 1/2 medium or 1/3 cup |
| Tomato | 1 large or 1 cup | Tomato sauce or puree | 1/2 cup |
| Juice: tomato or mixed vegetable | 1 cup | Tomato paste | 1/4 cup |
| | | Soups: tomato, vegetable, vegetable-meat (made with water) | 1/2 cup |

# MISCELLANEOUS FOODS EXCHANGE LIST
## (40 calories per exchange)

These foods and beverages provide concentrated sources of calories. The alcoholic beverages and most of the sweet foods supply calories without nutrients, *use them sparingly*.

**List 1. (Fats)** Each of these provides approximately 40 calories per exchange. Those in bold type are good sources of polyunsaturated fatty acids. Include some in your diet daily.

| | | | |
|---|---|---|---|
| Avocado | 1/8 4-inch diameter | Nuts | 6 small |
| Bacon, crisp | 1 slice | **Oil** (safflower, sunflower, corn, | 1 teaspoon |
| Butter, hard margarine, | 1 teaspoon | soybean, cottonseed) | |
| cooking fat | | Olives | 5 small |
| **Soft margarine** | 1 teaspoon | Sour cream | 2 tablespoons |
| **Cream cheese** | 1 tablespoon | Whipped cream | 1 rounded |
| **French dressing** | 1 tablespoon | | tablespoon |
| **Mayonnaise** | 1 teaspoon | | |

**List 2. (Sweets & Starches)** The following provide 40 calories per exchange.

| | | | |
|---|---|---|---|
| Cocoa (sweetened) | 1 level tablespoon | Sugar, syrup, honey, jam, jelly | 1 level tablespoon |
| Hard candy (small) or | 1 | Flour, corn starch | 1 rounded |
| caramel | | | tablespoon |

**List 3. (Desserts and beverages)** These foods, in the amounts specified, supply approximately 80 calories and must be counted as 2 miscellaneous food exchanges.

| Desserts | | | |
|---|---|---|---|
| | | Any dessert, if 1 serving | 1 serving |
| Cake: sponge, angel food | 1 piece, 2 x 2 x 1 inches | portion is no more than 80 calories | |
| | | Beverages . | |
| Jello | 1 serving (5 per package) | Beer, carbonated beverages | 6 ounces |
| | | Wine (light, dry) | 3 ounces |
| Sherbet, ice milk, ice cream | 1/3 cup | | |

# Appendix B
# **Food Calorie Plans**

## 1200–CALORIE FOOD PLAN

**EXCHANGES**

| | 6<br>MEAT | 4<br>GRAIN | 2<br>MILK | 5<br>FRUIT & VEG | 3<br>MISC |
|---|---|---|---|---|---|
| **MORNING** | ☐ | ☐ | ☐ | ☐ | ☐ |
| **AFTERNOON** | ☐ ☐ | ☐ ☐ | ☐ | ☐ | ☐ |
| **EVENING** | ☐ ☐ ☐ | ☐ | | ☐ ☐ ☐ | ☐ |
| **OTHER FOODS** | | | | | |

| FOOD PLAN TOTAL | EXTRAS | TOTAL CALORIES |
|---|---|---|
| | | |

# 1350–CALORIE FOOD PLAN

EXCHANGES

|  | 6<br>MEAT | 5<br>GRAIN | 2<br>MILK | 6<br>FRUIT & VEG | 4<br>MISC |
|---|---|---|---|---|---|
| MORNING | ☐ | ☐ ☐ | ☐ | ☐ | ☐ |
| AFTERNOON | ☐ ☐ | ☐ ☐ | ☐ | ☐ ☐ | ☐ ☐ |
| EVENING | ☐ ☐ ☐ | ☐ | | ☐ ☐ ☐ | ☐ |
| OTHER<br>FOODS | | | | | |

| FOOD PLAN TOTAL | EXTRAS | TOTAL CALORIES |
|---|---|---|

# 1500-CALORIE FOOD PLAN

EXCHANGES

| | 6 MEAT | 6 GRAIN | 2 MILK | 7 FRUIT & VEG | 5 MISC |
|---|---|---|---|---|---|
| MORNING | ☐ ☐ | ☐ ☐ | ☐ | ☐ ☐ | ☐ ☐ |
| AFTERNOON | ☐ ☐ | ☐ ☐ ☐ | ☐ | ☐ ☐ | ☐ ☐ |
| EVENING | ☐ ☐ ☐ ☐ | ☐ | | ☐ ☐ ☐ | ☐ |
| OTHER FOODS | | | | | |

| FOOD PLAN TOTAL | EXTRAS | TOTAL CALORIES |
|---|---|---|
| | | |

# 1700—CALORIE FOOD PLAN
EXCHANGES

| | 7 MEAT | 7 GRAIN | 2 MILK | 7 FRUIT & VEG | 6 MISC |
|---|---|---|---|---|---|
| MORNING | ☐ | ☐ | ☐ | ☐ | ☐ |
| | | ☐ | | ☐ | ☐ |
| | | ☐ | | | |
| AFTERNOON | ☐ | ☐ | ☐ | ☐ | ☐ |
| | ☐ | ☐ | | ☐ | ☐ |
| | | ☐ | | | |
| EVENING | ☐ | ☐ | | ☐ | ☐ |
| | ☐ | | | ☐ | ☐ |
| | ☐ | | | ☐ | |
| | ☐ | | | | |
| OTHER FOODS | | | | | |

| FOOD PLAN TOTAL | EXTRAS | TOTAL CALORIES |
|---|---|---|
| | | |

© Research Press Company

# 1900–CALORIE FOOD PLAN

EXCHANGES

|  | 7<br>MEAT | 8<br>GRAIN | 3<br>MILK | 7<br>FRUIT & VEG | 7<br>MISC |
|---|---|---|---|---|---|
| MORNING | ☐ | ☐ | ☐ | ☐ | ☐ |
|  |  | ☐ |  | ☐ | ☐ |
|  |  | ☐ |  |  |  |
| AFTERNOON | ☐ | ☐ | ☐ | ☐ | ☐ |
|  | ☐ | ☐ |  | ☐ | ☐ |
|  |  | ☐ |  |  |  |
| EVENING | ☐ | ☐ | ☐ | ☐ | ☐ |
|  | ☐ | ☐ |  | ☐ | ☐ |
|  | ☐ |  |  | ☐ | ☐ |
|  | ☐ |  |  |  |  |
| OTHER FOODS |  |  |  |  |  |

| FOOD PLAN TOTAL | EXTRAS | TOTAL CALORIES |
|---|---|---|
|  |  |  |

# 2100–CALORIE FOOD PLAN
EXCHANGES

| | 7 MEAT | 9 GRAIN | 3 MILK | 8 FRUIT & VEG | 9 MISC |
|---|---|---|---|---|---|
| **MORNING** | ☐ | ☐ | ☐ | ☐ | ☐ |
| | | ☐ | | ☐ | ☐ |
| | | ☐ | | | |
| **AFTERNOON** | ☐ | ☐ | ☐ | ☐ | ☐ |
| | ☐ | ☐ | | ☐ | ☐ |
| | | ☐ | | | ☐ |
| **EVENING** | ☐ | ☐ | ☐ | ☐ | ☐ |
| | ☐ | ☐ | | ☐ | ☐ |
| | ☐ | ☐ | | ☐ | ☐ |
| | ☐ | | | ☐ | ☐ |
| **OTHER FOODS** | | | | | |

| FOOD PLAN TOTAL | EXTRAS | TOTAL CALORIES |
|---|---|---|
| | | |

# 2300—CALORIE FOOD PLAN

EXCHANGES

| 8 MEAT | 10 GRAIN | 3 MILK | 8 FRUIT & VEG | 11 MISC |
|--------|----------|--------|---------------|---------|

**MORNING**

**AFTERNOON**

**EVENING**

**OTHER FOODS**

| FOOD PLAN TOTAL | EXTRAS | TOTAL CALORIES |
|-----------------|--------|----------------|

© Research Press Company

# PERSONALIZED FOOD PLAN

EXCHANGES

| | MEAT | GRAIN | MILK | FRUIT & VEG | MISC |
|---|---|---|---|---|---|
| MORNING | | | | | |
| AFTERNOON | | | | | |
| EVENING | | | | | |
| OTHER FOODS | | | | | |

| FOOD PLAN TOTAL | EXTRAS | TOTAL CALORIES |
|---|---|---|
| | | |

© Research Press Company

# Appendix C
# **Exercise Plan** *

| LIGHT EXERCISE | |
|---|---|
| | Each box = 5 min. = 20 calories |
| | x20= |
| MODERATE EXERCISE | |
| | Each box = 5 min. = 35 calories |
| | x35= |
| HEAVY EXERCISE | |
| | Each box = 5 min. = 50 calories |
| | x50= |
| **DAILY TOTAL** | |

*Caloric values are for gross energy expenditure.

© Research Press Company

# Appendix D
# Daily Eating, Exercise, and Weight Control Graph

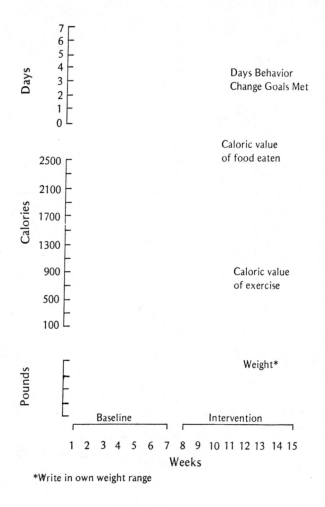

*Write in own weight range

# Appendix E
# **Daily Eating Record Form**

Date:

Circle the Day:

Monday Tuesday Wednesday Thursday Friday Saturday Sunday

| Hour | Did you eat: | | | Did you feel: | | | Were you: | | | Where were you? | | | What were you doing? | | |
|------|--------------|--|--|---------------|--|--|-----------|--|--|-----------------|--|--|----------------------|--|--|
| | Nothing | As planned | Not as planned | Relaxed | Tired | Tense | Alone | With family | With friends | Home | Work | Visiting restaurant | Work | Active | Inactive |
| 7:00 | | | | | | | | | | | | | | | |
| 8:00 | | | | | | | | | | | | | | | |
| 9:00 | | | | | | | | | | | | | | | |
| 10:00 | | | | | | | | | | | | | | | |
| 11:00 | | | | | | | | | | | | | | | |
| 12:00 | | | | | | | | | | | | | | | |
| 1:00 | | | | | | | | | | | | | | | |
| 2:00 | | | | | | | | | | | | | | | |
| 3:00 | | | | | | | | | | | | | | | |

154

Date:

Circle the Day:

Monday  Tuesday  Wednesday  Thursday  Friday  Saturday  Sunday

| Hour | Did you eat: | | | Did you feel: | | | Were you: | | | Where were you? | | | What were you doing? | | |
|---|---|---|---|---|---|---|---|---|---|---|---|---|---|---|---|
| | Nothing | As planned | Not as planned | Relaxed | Tired | Tense | Alone | With family | With friends | Home | Work | Visiting restaurant | Work | Active | Inactive |
| 4:00 | | | | | | | | | | | | | | | |
| 5:00 | | | | | | | | | | | | | | | |
| 6:00 | | | | | | | | | | | | | | | |
| 7:00 | | | | | | | | | | | | | | | |
| 8:00 | | | | | | | | | | | | | | | |
| 9:00 | | | | | | | | | | | | | | | |
| 10:00 | | | | | | | | | | | | | | | |
| 11:00 | | | | | | | | | | | | | | | |
| 12:00 | | | | | | | | | | | | | | | |

# Appendix F
# **Mean Energy Expenditure of Various Activities**

The values are expressed in calories/minute of gross body expenditure.

|   |   | Body weight, pounds | Calories*/ minute |
|---|---|---|---|
| 1. | Personal necessities | | |
| | Sitting, eating | 143 | 1.5 |
| | Washing and dressing | 150 | 1.2 |
| | | 150 | 2.6 |
| 2. | Locomotion | | |
| | Cycling, 5.5 mph | 156 | 4.5 |
| | Cycling, 9.4 mph | 156 | 7.0 |
| | Cycling, 13.1 mph | 156 | 11.1 |
| | Driving a car | 141 | 2.8 |
| | Walking, 2 mph | 160 | 3.2 |
| | Walking, 3 mph | 160 | 4.4 |
| | Walking, 4 mph | 160 | 5.8 |
| | Walking downstairs | 161 | 7.1 |
| | Walking upstairs | 161 | 18.6 |
| 3. | Sedentary occupations | | |
| | Classwork, lecture | 150 | 1.7 |
| | Sitting, reading | 161 | 1.3 |
| | Standing, light activity | 161 | 2.6 |
| | Typing, 40 words/min., mechanical typewriter | 121 | 1.7 |
| | Typing, 40 words/min., electric typewriter | 121 | 1.5 |
| 4. | Domestic work | | |
| | Bed making | 121 | 3.5 |
| | Dusting | 121 | 2.5 |
| | Ironing | 121 | 1.7 |
| | Preparing a meal | 121 | 2.5 |
| | Scrubbing floors | 121 | 4.0 |
| | Shopping with heavy load | 121 | 4.0 |
| | Window cleaning | 121 | 3.5 |
| 5. | Light industry | | |
| | Assembly work in car factory | 121 | 2.3 |
| | Carpentry | 150 | 3.8 |

|  | | |
|---|---|---|
| Farming chores | 150 | 3.8 |
| Farming, haying, plowing with horse | 150 | 6.7 |
| House painting | 150 | 3.5 |
| Metal working | 150 | 3.5 |
| Mixing cement | 150 | 4.7 |
| Stone, masonry | 150 | 6.3 |
| Truck and automobile repair | 150 | 4.2 |

**6. Heavy work**

| | | |
|---|---|---|
| Dragging logs | 143 | 12.1 |
| Drilling coal or rock | 143 | 6.1 |
| Felling trees | 143 | 8.6 |
| Gardening, digging | 139 | 8.6 |
| Pick and shovel work | 143 | 8.6 |

**7. Recreation**

| | | |
|---|---|---|
| Canoeing, 2.5 mph | 150 | 3.0 |
| Canoeing, 4 mph | 150 | 7.0 |
| Cross country running | 143 | 10.6 |
| Dancing, waltz | 167 | 5.2 |
| Dancing, rumba | 152 | 5.7 |
| Golfing | 139 | 5.0 |
| Gymnastics exercises: | | |
|   Balancing exercises | 150 | 2.5 |
|   Trunk bending | 150 | 3.5 |
| Mountain climbing | 150 | 10.0 |
| Playing baseball (except pitcher) | 150 | 4.7 |
| Playing basketball | 161 | 8.6 |
| Playing football (American) | 161 | 10.2 |
| Playing pingpong | 161 | 4.9 |
| Playing tennis | 154 | 7.1 |
| Playing squash | 147 | 10.2 |
| Playing volleyball | 150 | 3.5 |
| Skiing, level hard snow, moderate speed | 125 | 10.8 |
| Skiing, up hill hard snow, maximum speed | 150 | 18.6 |
| Sprinting | 150 | 23.3 |
| Snowshoeing, 2.27 mph | 150 | 6.2 |

*The calorie used in human metabolism is the heat needed to raise the temperature of one kilogram (2.2 pounds) of water from 15 degrees to 16 degrees Centigrade.

Adapted from the following:
J. V. G. A. Durnin and R. Passmore. *Energy, work and leisure.* London: Heinemann Educational Books Ltd., 1967. Pp. 49, 57, 72, 76.

R. Passmore and J. V. G. A. Durnin. Human energy expenditure. *Physiological Reviews,* 1955, *35,* 811-813.

C. F. Consolazio, R. E. Johnson, and I. J. Pecora. *Physiological measurements of metabolic functions in man.* New York: McGraw-Hill, 1963. Pp. 330-332.

# Appendix G
# **Equivalents by Volume**

(All measurements level)

| | |
|---|---|
| 1 quart | = 4 cups |
| 1 cup | = 8 fluid ounces |
| | = ½ pint |
| | = 16 tablespoons |
| | |
| 2 tablespoons | = 1 fluid ounce |
| 1 tablespoon | = 3 teaspoons |
| 1 pound regular butter or margarine | = 4 sticks |
| | = 2 cups |
| | |
| 1 pound whipped butter or margarine | = 6 sticks |
| | = 2  8-ounce containers |
| | = 3 cups |

# Notes

Where will you plan to eat?

What activities will you be careful to avoid while eating?

What are the times of your weaknesses during the eating day?

What steps can you take to change them?

How can you improve your eating habits?

## ABOUT THE AUTHOR

Dr. Richard B. Stuart is Professor of Psychology and Social Work at the University of Utah. He is also Psychological Director of Weight Watchers International. He has in the past held professorships at the University of Michigan and the University of British Columbia. He is Past President of the Association for Advancement of Behavior Therapy and a Fellow of the American Psychological Association. He has written six books and over 90 professional journal articles. Dr. Stuart's pioneering research in the behavioral control of overeating has helped to stimulate over 200 independent evaluations of these techniques.

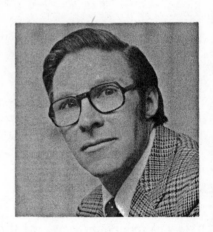

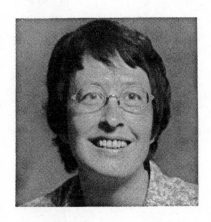

## ABOUT THE AUTHOR

Barbara Davis has had extensive experience in the field of nutrition. Her work has ranged from the planning and evaluation of nutrition and exercise programs on the North American continent to the training of nutrition personnel in the Third World. Mrs. Davis completed her undergraduate work at the University of British Columbia and received her Masters degree in Nutritional Science from the University of Michigan. While at the University of Michigan she worked as a lecturer and research assistant and as a nutrition consultant for both individual and group weight-control programs. Mrs. Davis has recently spent three years in Africa and was involved in training nutrition extension workers. On her return to North America she worked as a research nutritionist at the Toronto Western Hospital Weight Control Clinic, University of Toronto, and continues to act as consultant to that Clinic. She is presently employed in the field of community nutrition. Mrs. Davis is a member of the Society for Nutrition Education and the Society of Nutritionists and Public Health.